That You May Live Long

That You
May Live Long

Caring for Our Aging Parents,
Caring for Ourselves

RICHARD F. ADDRESS

and HARA E. PERSON

UAHC Press • New York, New York

The Publisher would like to gratefully acknowledge the following for granting permission to reprint previously published material:

KLUWER ACADEMIC/PLENUM PUBLISHERS: "Jewish Values and Sociopsychological Perspectives on Aging" by Dr. Robert L. Katz from *Pastoral Psychology* 24, no. 229 (winter 1975); "Who Pays? The Talmudic Approach to Filial Responsibility" by Michael Chernick from *The Journal of Aging and Judaism* 1, no. 2 (spring/summer 1987). Reprinted by permission of Kluwer Academic/Plenum Publishers.

RUTH LANGER: "Honor Your Father and Mother: Caregiving as a Halakhic Responsibility" by Ruth Langer from *Aging and the Aged in Jewish Law* edited by Walter Jacob and Moshe Zemer. Reprinted by permission of Ruth Langer.

Library of Congress Cataloging-in-Publication Data

That you may live long : caring for our aging parents, caring for ourselves / [edited by] Richard F. Address and Hara E. Person.
    p. cm.
    Includes bibliographical references.
    ISBN 0-8074-0792-5 (pbk. : alk. paper)
    1. Aging parents—Care—Religious aspects—Judaism. 2. Parent and adult child—United States. 3. Caregivers—Family relationships—United States. I. Address, Richard F. II. Person, Hara.

HQ1063.6.T48 2003
306.874'0846—dc21   2002023962

For my grandmother, Augusta Goetz, z"l,
in loving memory.
—HEP

To all those who find the strength and spirit to fulfill
the call of the Fifth Commandment. May you continue
to go from strength to strength.
—RFA

And for all the parents, grandparents, and loved ones
whose lives inspired the essays in this book.

Honor your father and your mother,
that you may live long on the land
that *Adonai* your God is giving you.

—Exodus 20:12

Note on Translations

Many of the authors included in this volume have used different translations of the same texts in their essays. The editors have chosen to keep the variations in translation as indicated by the authors.

Acknowledgments

⚜

The thoughts and experiences of many people went into the creation of this book. We would have liked all of those who submitted essays to be included in the collection and regret that we were not able to use them all. All the essays that were submitted helped us understand more about our topic, and we are grateful for each submission.

We would both like to thank our departments at the UAHC, who helped in the creation of this book in a variety of ways. From the Department of Jewish Family Concerns, we would like to express our gratitude to Marcia Hochman, assistant director of the department, and likewise to Lynn Levy and Anthony Selvitella. The department's leadership has been a source of great support, and so we thank our chair, Jean Abarbanel, as well as vice-chairs Mike Grunebaum and Steve Picheny. Finally, many members of the Department of Jewish Family Concerns and colleagues helped shape this book, including Steve Burkett, Davna Brook, Susan Bortz, Harriet Rosen, Dr. James Soffer, Janice Bergman, Rabbi Jonathan Kendall, Laura Sperling, Rabbi Alan Fuchs, and Rabbi Oren Postrel.

From the UAHC Press, we owe enormous thanks to Ken Gesser, who agreed that there was a need for such a book and encouraged us at every step of the way; Stuart Benick, for his bookmaking know-how; and Rick Abrams, for his commitment to this book. We owe many thanks to Liane Broido, who was invaluable in helping with the organization and assembling of the book; Eric Eisenkramer, for taking a thorough look at the manuscript in its early stages; Jeremy Master, for creating the bibliography; and Debra Hirsch Corman, who patiently helped to give the book its final shape and knew all the right questions to ask.

Much work, effort, and time goes into creating a book. We would like to warmly thank all of those who helped, encouraged, and supported us, including Dr. Diane Person, Stanley Person, Yigal Rechtman, Liya Rechtman, Yoni Rechtman, Dr. Kerry Olitzky, and Dr. Adina Kalet. A special thank-you also goes to the extended Rechtman and Marcus clan, for allowing their photograph of a four-generation family group to be used on the cover.

The impetus for this book came originally from Hara's experience in helping her mother, Diane Person, deal with the illness and related care of her grandmother, Augusta Goetz. It was during that period that the need for such a book first became clear. Luckily, when Richie was approached with the idea of collaborating on such a book, having worked for many years on issues connected to aging and caregiving, he was enthusiastic and ready to begin. The collaboration has been a wonderful experience, and for this blessing of working together we are particularly thankful.

Contents

ᥴᘐ ᘘᕽ

Acknowledgments xi

Introduction: Celebrating the Art of Caregiving
RABBI RICHARD F. ADDRESS 1

Caring for Our Parents, Caring for Ourselves:
A Jewish Perspective
DR. ALBERT MICAH LEWIS 9

Death Is Inevitable, but Being Prepared Isn't
ᘘᕽ Harriet H. Rosen 15

Caring for Our Parents by Making Decisions Together
RABBI THOMAS A. LOUCHHEIM 21

Growing Old Isn't for the Faint of Heart: Making Decisions Together
ᘘᕽ Rabbi Jonathan P. Kendall 34

Jewish Values and Sociopsychological Perspectives on Aging
DR. ROBERT L. KATZ, *z"l* 45

Spiritual Aging
RABBI JACK STERN   62

Five Women Spanning Four Generations
ॐ   Rabbi David Wolfman   68

Beyond Guilt: What We Owe Our Aging Parents—
A Perspective from Tradition
RABBI DAYLE A. FRIEDMAN   78

Honor Thy Mother and Thy Father
ॐ   Janice London Bergman   90

Who Pays? The Talmudic Approach to Filial Responsibility
RABBI MICHAEL CHERNICK   94

The Psychodynamics of Caring for Aging Parents
RABBI DEBORAH PIPE-MAZO   103

Becoming an Expert on the Individual, Not the Disease
ॐ   Kathryn Kahn   108

Honor Your Father and Mother:
Caregiving as a Halachic Responsibility
RABBI RUTH LANGER   113

The Gift of a Lifetime
ॐ   Laura Sperling   127

A Jewish Way of Thinking about Nursing Homes
RABBI SHELDON MARDER   131

When Our Parents Can No Longer Decide
RABBI SANDRA ROSENTHAL BERLINER   139

A Granddaughter's Story: One Family's Decision-Making Process
🙠 Dr. Adina Kalet 147

On Suffering
RABBI ALAN HENKIN 158

When the Time Came
🙠 Dr. James Soffer 167

Accepting Death: The Caregiver's Dilemma
RABBI W. GUNTHER PLAUT 171

Letting the Cycle of Life Do Its Work: The Miracle of Death
🙠 Rabbi Hara E. Person 176

Notes 180

Suggested Reading 191

Contributors 193

That You May Live Long

Introduction:
Celebrating the Art of Caregiving

RABBI RICHARD F. ADDRESS

Sitting again in the waiting room of a hospital. Waiting with a parent to see another doctor. Making idle conversation and flashing back on so many moments in life when situations were reversed. No matter how prepared for such moments you think you are, the reality of caregiving challenges much of what we take for granted, daring us to examine our priorities. Often unspoken in the moments when the parent-child relationship is reversed is the motif of Genesis 3: our confrontation with mortality and our need to see this in terms of something greater than ourselves.

The realization that the caregiving equation within the parent-child relationship has shifted emerges in ways that reflect the uniqueness of life's randomness. Slowly, like shifting sands that restructure a favorite patch of beach—or suddenly, as in the late-night phone call from a parent's friend that informs you of news you have always feared—new realities reconfigure what had been routine. The challenges presented to so many of us in caring for our aging parents test the basic relationships of parent and child and, if we allow it, can open up new pathways to meaning and understanding. These are often moments that test us. These are also moments in which the mystery of God's presence can be present to provide a reservoir of strength, faith, and spiritual growth. One thing is true: few people are ever the same after assuming the role of caregiver.

This book is an attempt to present insights into the art of caregiving. It does so from two perspectives: the Jewish texts and personal experiences. We have intertwined the text-based essays and the personal reflections in order to highlight how theory is put into practice. These reflections illustrate a variety of circumstances and reactions to the challenge of caregiving. What does emerge from these reflections is a life-affirming reaction to what they, as adult children, have been called upon to do. Throughout situations that require restructuring of family concerns, emotional and financial sacrifice, one theme remains constant. There is an implicit understanding that in taking care of a parent, you are modeling behavior observed when you were a child. Rabbi Jack Stern alludes to this powerful generational gift when he writes of the sacred act of "giving back" to our parents what they gave to us and to others.

The world in which we live has created a new life-cycle stage, the caregiver. This contemporary category of life, often lasting for years, may be coupled with membership in another of our society's new roles, the so-called "sandwich generation." As those of us who are living this life will attest, and as the personal reflections will confirm, the sandwich is often multilayered, and the stresses and strains often pull in opposite directions. For many, the casualty in all of this may be our own "self." For many of us, this new life stage is a tenuous balancing act between duties, obligations, guilts, fears, hopes, and dreams. How the organized Jewish community in general and the synagogue community in particular respond to these very real concerns will go a long way in determining the type of community we create and the style of caring that we model. We cannot forget that despite the rise of and need for "facilities" and other caregiving institutions, our children will watch and learn how to do this for our loved ones just as we observed our parents when we were young.

Embracing this behavior is the pull and power and passion of the sacred relationships that have been formed over a lifetime. It is these relationships that form the practical theology of caregiving.

The foundation for our actions in the area of caregiving is the classic texts of Torah that implore us to "honor and respect" our parents. The commandment appears three times in Torah: Exodus 20:12 and Deuteronomy 5:16, where we are commanded to "honor" (*kabeid*) our father and mother; and Leviticus 19:3, where we are commanded to *tira-u*, "revere" or "respect" our mother and father. The midrash reminds us that the two orders, father/mother and mother/father, appear to insure that no parent receives special attention, that both are treated equally.

This injunction is met in the daily prayer book, in which we are reminded that honoring our parents is an action whose reward is without measure. A commentary on Proverbs 3:9 that parallels honoring parents with honoring God says that we honor through our financial resources as well as material and psychological resources. Yet, the tradition is clear that the family is not required to impoverish themselves in the pursuit of fulfilling the commandment. Parents have a responsibility to handle as much of their own financial obligations of caregiving as possible. The exploration of these texts and the development of several interpretations form the basis of several of the text-based articles that appear here. Rabbis Ruth Langer and Michael Chernick take us through a variety of interpretations and nuances that have great relevance in today's world.

Especially important are the discussions as to how far a child can or should be expected to go in taking care of a parent when that caregiving may impact on the well-being of the caregiver and the caregiver's own family. These include the psychological and economic issues that are present in so many of our family situations today, which were anticipated in the commentaries. Langer and Chernick also allude to other contemporary concerns that deal with the emotions felt when a child must take care of a parent with whom there was less than a healthy relationship. That raises the issue of whether one assumes the responsibility for caregiving out of a sense of love or, as Jewish tradition teaches, out of a response to a divine call, obligation, and duty. Dr. Robert L. Katz *(z"l)*, who taught at Hebrew Union College, places much of this in another profound context in his classic essay on the use of empathy in caring.

The link between how we take care of loved ones and our relationship with God is an often neglected and much denied subtlety of the caregiving experience. That is why the texts so strongly stress the idea of respecting our loved one's wishes. In a society of rapidly developing medical technology, this idea of respecting a loved one's wishes can create tension when those wishes may conflict with our own. Part of caregiving in the twenty-first century is taking the time to discuss openly what people want, under what circumstances, and why. Dr. Albert Micah Lewis alludes to the fact that those discussions may need to be the open and honest exchange of differing points of view. The time to have those discussions is when all parties can participate. This is now a modern mitzvah. Rabbi Thomas A. Louchheim expands this reality in urging the need for communication and education in dealing with our loved ones. The "mitzvah" of honoring and respecting a parent's wishes takes on real perspective in the reflections of Dr. James Soffer and Janice London Bergman, who each dealt with honor and respect of parental wishes from their own perspectives. They remind us that the difficulties of certain caregiving situations are understandable only through personal experience. A lesson that emerges from all of the personal reflections is that there may be *no* template for taking care of someone. The midrash is correct when it reminds us that each person is unique and thus each caring situation will be as well.

Rabbis Dayle A. Freidman and Deborah Pipe-Mazo take us through discussions that reflect some of the personal and psychological tensions that are created in caregiving. The desire to "do what is right" versus the fear that "I will not be able to" is often a reality. We are reminded that this tension is often the product of the shifting roles that emerge during the caregiving process. These different and often fluid stages that we pass through give rise to a variety of emotions that can overwhelm us like waves in rapid fashion. Rabbi W. Gunther Plaut alludes to the fact that we often do not know what to pray for, as the range of emotions can be so great. Dr. Adina Kalet and Kathy Kahn write with an intensity born from experience on the myriad of emotions that confront the caregiver in trying to make sense of this new life stage. Conflicting emotions and the desire for some sense of meaning are constant companions.

A continuing issue that confronts families and caregivers is how to begin to make sacred decisions regarding loved ones when they cannot speak for themselves or when the reality emerges that independent living is no longer possible. Rabbis Sandra Rosenthal Berliner and Sheldon Marder take us through some of the difficulties and challenges that need to be negotiated in these all too common situations. How can one begin to decide when and where a loved one needs to be placed in a caregiving facility? What is the role of hospice care in our dialogues? How can one balance family, distance, and one's own emotions in such situations? Laura Sperling and Rabbi Jonathan P. Kendall reflect on their particular journeys of placing a loved one in a caregiving facility. Again, as with all the selections in this volume, Jewish tradition and texts can be instructive in guiding us through the possibilities of decision making.

Finally, Rabbi Hara Person writes of the difficult path that her family took in the care of her grandmother. It is a path that encompasses many of the personal testimonies within this book. The journey includes stages of how the anger associated with the reality of her grandmother's situation progressed from a search for meaning within the suffering to the acceptance on the part of her family to allow "the cycle of life to do its work." Anger and questioning evolved to meaning through acceptance, the meaning embraced by an ethic of sacred personal relationships.

Many of the discussions that take place within the contexts of the essays and reflections touch on the dilemma of trying to make sense of out suffering. Rabbi Alan Henkin deals with this issue with care and sensitivity, reminding us that we do not seek to suffer, but that is a part of our being alive, and how we choose to deal with it helps to shape how we choose to be in the image and likeness of God. Part of taking these events into our own soul is the difficulty in understanding the concept of "letting go." Harriet Rosen reflects on this when she writes of her journey with her father, reminding us that while death may be inevitable, our being prepared is not.

The personal reflections, as a whole, affirm the value of life and the powerful opportunities that present themselves for sacred moments. There is a sense of life's preciousness and the need to be open to lessons that can be learned and passed on through the many generations. Rabbi David Wolfman writes of this in his reflection on life with several generations of people within his own home. The lessons learned from involvement in multigenerational caregiving speak to another underlying reality that emerges from these essays and reflections. That is the ultimate power of creating sacred personal relationships. Throughout the contents of this volume is the reality that success in caregiving, whatever that may mean, is not primarily based on the acquisition of specific knowledge; rather, success is based on the level and power of the relationship that are established within the caregiving experience. Being there, holding a hand, sitting in that waiting room or nursing home may be, ultimately, as powerful as any medication. Bringing God's presence into the present becomes a mitzvah the reward for which really is without measure and, as is demonstrated in the personal reflections, is equally powerful for both caregiver and the person receiving the care.

As you examine the essays and reflections in this volume, remember that we have de facto created a new life-cycle stage in our life's journey.

The caregiver, often sandwiched among many generations, is a reality of everyday life that will continue. Often, these individuals struggle in isolation, stressed and overwhelmed by trying to do what is right, often at great physical, emotional, spiritual, and economic cost. For many congregations and communities, creative programs of support have already been developed, and variations on this caring community theme are in constant evolution. Yet, let us make one additional suggestion. Given the realities of our society, the time may be at hand for congregations and communities to create ceremonies, rituals, and occasions on which caregivers may be honored.

We suggest the creation of a new category of honor within our community, the *shomeir*. The word means "guardian" and, in many ways, "a caretaker." It is time for us to honor these people, to celebrate what they do and the sacrifices they make to fulfill the Fifth Commandment. They are living the concept of *dugmah*, "example," for the community, their families, and the future. In honoring the *shomeir*, we would give recognition to the various aspects that characterize living in the middle: the ability to care for a loved one and the necessity of caring for one's self. We need to find a way not only to honor the giving of care to another, but of reminding the person who gives that taking care of one's self is equally important. This is the other side of the caregiving coin that is so often forgotten, the side that so often leads to feelings of depression and family crises. Susan Bortz of Pittsburgh wrote of this double-sided tension within her own multigenerational experience: "The obligation to honor our parents may weigh heavy on our shoulders and our souls, as is balancing our responsibilities and our time with and for all members of our families. The balancing act takes careful planning, and should include an obligation to take care of one's self and should be a part of a routine so one does not neglect or forget time with family, prayer, study, and exercise."[1]

Caregiving, as the personal reflections illustrate, can place overwhelming stresses on one's own emotional, physical, and spiritual health. It may be time for us to institutionalize, through programs, rituals, and events, this new life stage: the caregiver.

As Laura Sperling writes:

> I became trained to be my mother's nurse, business manager, and aggressive advocate. I administered every manner of med-

ication, including intravenous hydrations and medicines. Yet, despite the long hours and complex challenges, the ability to be there for my parents, especially my mother, over a continuous period of time was a profound sacrifice and gift that I could give to her. She certainly would have done that for me.

So may it be with us, that we may all live long.

Caring for Our Parents,
Caring for Ourselves:
A Jewish Perspective

DR. ALBERT MICAH LEWIS

Caring, as understood on the deepest of levels as that between God and the Jewish people, is a mutuality in which both the giver and the recipient benefit and each truly loves and needs the other. In an ideal world, parents and children, grandparents, grandchildren, and other family members would love, respect, care for, and encourage one another. Cain's question to God, "Am I my brother's keeper?" (Genesis 4:9), would be returned with a resounding, "Yes, and your sister's and your parents' and your entire extended family's!" Unfortunately, we do not live in a perfect world, and until the messianic age arrives, we will have to struggle with conflicts of time, personality, interests, and even money. The aging of America and the increased emotional (and sometimes physical and financial) responsibilities often placed on middle-aged children and their families add stress to an already stressful life. Caregiving, whether by a young mother to her baby or by a middle-aged son to his aging father, can be both rewarding and exhausting. Fortunately, Jewish tradition has wrestled with this dilemma for well over four thousand years and can guide us in how and when to set limits, recognize responsibilities, and take care of ourselves at the same time.

For families caught in the dilemma of giving care to their parents while trying to maintain a normal life, it may be helpful to take another look at the biblical injunction "Honor your father and your mother *that your days may be long upon the land that* Adonai *your God is giving you*" (Exodus 20:12). Like other biblical laws, this commandment was developed to address a specific need. It is not a natural instinct for children to give care to their aging parents. Even in the biblical period, adult children must have struggled with the demands of their own lives and families, demands that were no less and probably even greater than ours. The community realized that the abandonment of the aged must be addressed and that communally sanctioned law must be developed. The fifth commandment—"Honor your father and your mother"—is the resulting law. It teaches that even though this kind of caregiving may not feel natural or even fair, it must be provided. In a later period, the prophets would speak about the desolation that would be visited upon Israel if it did not properly care for its aged. In the Babylonian Talmud, the following stories are told:

> There are three partners in man: the Holy One, blessed be He, the father, and the mother. When a person honors his father and his mother, God says, "It is as though I had dwelt among them and they had honored Me."
>
> BT *Kiddushin* 30b

> Respect an old man who has lost his learning: remember that the fragments of the tablets broken by Moses were preserved alongside the new.
>
> BT *B'rachot* 8b

Hillel, the first-century Rabbi and scholar, wrote about personal, family, and community responsibilities. From his insights we may learn how to give and receive care. In *Pirkei Avot* 1:14, Hillel states:

> *If I am not for myself, who will be for me?*
> *If I am only for myself, what am I?*
> *If not now, when?*

For the caregiver, Hillel's insight is about more than selfishness and responsibility; it is about achieving a balance of self-care and the care of others. When finding ourselves caring for a parent, we may ask, "If I do not take care of myself and address my own basic needs of nourishment and physical and emotional care, who will do so, and *how will I be effective in the care of another?"* Hillel teaches us as caregivers to attend to our own needs, and as receivers of care to look beyond our own pain. In reality, both the caregiver and the one cared for are part of the "family," and both need appropriate care. For the one who is cared for, Hillel also offers important insights: "If I cannot adequately care for myself, I am obligated to allow another trusted person to assist me . . . but I must be aware of his or her personal needs and feelings also. And, I may not wait until the last minute to accept or enlist the help I need."

The talmudic authorities, in both the Palestinian and the Babylonian versions, ruled that children have a responsibility to see that their parents are fed and cared for. Issues of disagreement arose between the two schools, however, about who should pay for this care. The Palestinian Rabbis argued that children must support their impoverished parents even if the children themselves are poverty stricken (JT *Kiddushin,* 1:7). The Babylonian Rabbis argued that the money for such support should come from the estate or funds of the parents (BT *Kiddushin* 32a). Contemporary Jewish thought would tell us that while we are obligated to look out for the welfare of our parents, we may not impoverish our children or ourselves in the effort. The creation of Jewish social service agencies, Jewish homes for the aged, and even the Jewish hospice movement are designed to address the needs of aging parents without impoverishing—emotionally or financially—their children. Today, some larger congregations even have social workers on their staffs to assist families with a variety of family issues. Additionally, when adult children can establish joint checking accounts and power of attorney for fragile parents *in advance of crises,* much anguish can be minimized. Open communication and trust are essential in such planning and actions. Again, the wisdom of Hillel—"if not now, when?"—helps us to see the clearer path.

In his classic work, *Mishneh Torah,* the medieval philosopher Maimonides tells us, "The words of Torah heal the soul, not the body."[1] In my own experience as a congregational rabbi for thirty-one years and as a counselor, I have found that my very presence and willingness to read selected portions of Torah or Psalms have brought great solace to people afflicted with a wide variety of diseases. I could help minimize their feelings of despair and abandonment. While I could not offer physical healing, I could offer hope and human caring. From this we can learn the importance of active listening, the difference between caring about and caring for an individual, and the role of the physician, caring friend, and family.

Maimonides reminds us that often our loved ones tell us about their physical or emotional pain with no expectation of our curing their condition. What they want most is to be heard and to know that we care. Sometimes, a caring comment like "I know you are very uncomfortable, and I wish I could take away your pain" will help another to know that we are listening and caring.

Knowing the difference between seeing that someone receives the necessary care and providing that care ourselves can also help us as the caregiver. Maimonides instructs us that "one should select as attendants and caretakers those who can cheer up the patient. This is a must in every illness."[2] Both Maimonides and Hillel help us to see the important difference between providing direct care ourselves and seeing that appropriate care is provided by another. Such recognition may be particularly difficult for middle-aged children to accept or acknowledge, because it brings to the surface the conflict of "independence versus dependence."

As middle-aged children, we are often struggling with our own issues of independence and self-definition while at the same time seeing the increasing dependence of our parents, as well as our own eventual dependency. The recognition itself creates a normal internal conflict. Additionally, it forces us to recognize that sometimes we truly are more effective and more caring of our parents and of all others in the family when we arrange for a second party to provide the appropriate care.

The more we can involve the recipient of the care in the decision process about who will directly give the care (bathing, feeding, transporting to physicians, daily companionship), the more we empower that family member—and show honor and respect. But even when that involvement is not possible because of emotional or physical distance, we are obligated to see that appropriate care is provided.

A second area of conflict for caregivers is that of "morality versus mortality," in which middle-aged children become increasingly aware of the decline of the aging parent. At this point, religious and societal values often dictate that one "should care for and about" the aging parent. In the Jewish community, we are fortunate to have the guidance of Hillel, Maimonides, and the talmudic Rabbis regarding "how" to care for and about one's parents. None of us, however, is immune from the feelings of guilt that often surface, especially as parents decline and die. It is common to hear people say, "I should have stayed longer," "I should have listened instead of making suggestions," "I could have done more." Our tradition tells us that sometimes the expectations of others—and even of ourselves—are unrealistic. Even Moses had to learn the art of delegating authority and responsibility. Had he not heeded the advice of his father-in-law, Jethro, he would not have been able to lead the Jewish people and maintain his sense of self (Exodus 18:17–23).

This is truly a time for family members to talk and to share feelings of frustration and inadequacy. One of the ways in which we honor our parents is through the sharing of our feelings with our partners, siblings, rabbis, and other caring people. The aging parents may also bring up anger, guilt, and a variety of unresolved issues concerning the adult children and deceased relatives. At age eighty-six, my father has begun to confide in me about issues that happened over seventy years ago. I have learned about how he saved my grandfather from a suicide attempt during the Depression, how he still remembers that it took two days before the U.S. Navy could find and identify my uncle's body at Normandy, and why my father felt he was an embarrassment to my grandfather. As difficult as it may be for us, by listening without judgment we honor our parents.

A third area that challenges us as middle-aged caregivers is the "integration versus isolation" issue. Here we see two struggles taking place at the same time. First, we feel that we have just begun or finally reached a sense of personal, professional, and intellectual integration, while our parent is becoming more isolated. Secondly, we fear that as the demands for care and support intensify, we too may become isolated from our partners, friends, and the activities we find meaningful. Much of the research dealing with the middle-aged couple indicates that it is a time when people become more settled as individuals and as partners. These areas provide yet more opportunities for discussion with family and extended support systems like the Jewish communal social worker or rabbi.

For both the caregiver and the one who receives care, contemporary rabbi Hayim Halevy Donin tells us that we have a responsibility to act in an accountable manner with regard to our own health. He reminds us of the instruction in Deuteronomy in which we are told, "For your own sake, therefore, be most careful" (4:15) and "Take utmost care and watch yourself scrupulously" (4:9).[3] Rabbi Benjamin Blech has written, "Honoring one's parents is the most difficult mitzvah in Judaism."[4] If it were easy we would have no need for gerontologists and therapists, nor would our tradition wrestle with this one issue for over four thousand years. In the retelling of the Ten Commandments in the book of Deuteronomy (5:16), the text states:

> Honor your father and your mother, as *Adonai*, your God commanded you; that your days may be long, and that it may go well with you, upon the land that *Adonai*, your God gives you.

From this text we glean several insights. We see that the care of the elderly parents was an obligation, which also contained an intrinsic reward—personal long life in the Land of Israel. As we care for our parents, we show our children and even our children's children what caring and family and loving long-term relationships are all about. Our reward for caring for our parents may not literally be a long life in the Land of Israel, but rather a kind of immortality through the ongoing transmission of our Jewish values. In these ways we continue to perpetuate the values of countless generations and to insure the life of these values for generations to come.

Death Is Inevitable,
but Being Prepared Isn't

────────────────

～

Harriet H. Rosen

What seems like chance played an important role in the events and decisions that preceded my father's death. Eight years ago, at a Shabbat morning minyan, an announcement was made that Holy Blossom Temple was having a program on living wills. With three aging parents living far away, my husband and I decided we should go to the program.

Afterwards, inspired by the program, we visited and spoke with our parents. Within the next two months, we learned their wishes, and their living wills were completed. I had been reluctant to talk to them about death, but these turned out to be far easier conversations than I had expected, as each of them had already experienced so much loss.

They were raised in environments where Jewish values were a part of their daily experience, so talking about death from a Jewish perspective wasn't foreign to them. The rites and the attitudes I seek as alternatives to our very secular world were built into their thinking. These conversations gave us an understanding and emotional footing that would make later decisions easier. They saw the living wills and the discussions as protection against what they feared far more, a prolonged and painful death.

When I noticed that my father had been losing weight, I attributed his weight loss to poorly fitting dentures. Chewing was painful, and no adjustments helped. We tried liquid supplements, but they upset his stomach. He continued to lose weight. I asked about what his doctor said. "He talks nonsense," my mother told me. "He's an alarmist."

Bells should have gone off in my brain during the visits that followed. They didn't. About six months later, my sister called to tell me she was concerned. We flew to California to see my parents. At my husband's urging, we took my father to see his doctor. We sat in the doctor's small office, knee to knee, and he told us that my father was in the advanced stages of prostate cancer and probably had about three to four months to live.

I sat in shock and my father, at ninety-one, just sat there and looked at us. Had he known before? I'll never know. He just smiled at us as if he didn't hear the doctor's words. My father, with full command of his mind, sharp and savvy, just sat there. When I was growing up, my father crawled into bed with a head cold and demanded nursing care. His behavior was a family joke, and we never took his complaining seriously. But a terminal illness brought no response at all from him except denial.

We stayed with him awhile and tried talking to him, but he waved the doctor's words aside. We dropped him off at home and I walked on the beach, crying into the wind. I asked God the questions everyone asks and tried to find some reason, some answer. Nothing came except pain.

"Everyone dies," my father had told me for years when we talked about all the deaths he had seen, all the losses he had experienced. One of nine children, he had lost all his siblings. His favorite brother and sister had died in their early forties. Within a four- or five-year span, he lost five people he loved. As much as he said that he accepted death and gave me the reasons provided by his intensely observant background, he remained angry with God for the pain that loss brought. He never stopped believing strongly in Jewish values, but some part of him remained unreconciled to so many losses following so hard one on the other. He held God accountable.

That mixture of faith, respect for God's power, and anger at death was something I became more aware of as he grew older. At his first ever Reform service, when the entire congregation stood to say *Kaddish*, he pulled me down. I had no reason to say *Kaddish*, he told me. Tradition, the complexity of his responses, and the acknowledgment of his connection were all in that moment.

From that doctor's visit forward, he never acknowledged that he was ill. We talked about death and dying, but never his. I tried tentatively a few times but met a solid wall of resistance. I talked to my mother, and she said not to discuss his impending death with him. I talked to my rabbi, who told me to honor my father's wishes. What I needed or thought I needed wasn't necessarily what he needed. So I honored his choice, but I remain unclear about whether that difficult choice was right. I think now how many things I'd like to know that I won't—ever.

My mother and I discussed his prognosis, and I told my sister about the doctor visit. They scarcely believed me. None of us seemed to have grasped the obvious. That he was ill, thin, and his color bad we could see, but the reality that he was failing rapidly didn't seem to connect with the signs we saw. We did, however, start to make decisions based on what we already knew my father wanted.

My mother and I talked to the doctor, and we arranged for the local hospice to provide my parents with support. Since we had already discussed the issue of no heroic measures, without which the California hospice will not participate, that step was a straightforward one. My parents signed the necessary papers and set the process in motion.

The hospice program provided a social worker who was assigned to my parents, and she visited regularly. Eight hours of home care made a bridge for my mother. It allowed her to use their resources slowly and, since my father died within a relatively short time, didn't deplete them.

Trained hospice volunteers came to visit with my father and give my mother time to herself. The primary caretaker, my mother, was herself seventy-nine years old. She was too old and too quickly drained physically and emotionally to manage the steadily more demanding tasks as my father's condition rapidly worsened. I arranged for more support and help.

I understand now the ways we each coped with his dying. I did things; I organized and called and looked for solutions. If I did enough, he wouldn't die. My mother made him food and became angry at his continually diminished appetite. If he would eat, he'd live. I explained that cancer eats too and that forcing him to eat wasn't good for him. She finally accepted my and the social worker's explanation. I wish someone had told me that the drive to do was just as useless.

So we waited. I found my heart hurt from the pain of waiting. I called my rabbi, and he listened to my grief. He told me the famous midrash about the students whose prayers kept an honored rabbi alive and the servant who allowed him to die by throwing a jug off the roof and interrupting their prayers. "Let go," he told me, "you must let go of those you love and allow them to leave." The thought was unbearable, but the reasoning was inescapable. He helped me understand my mother's reactions, and she and I talked about them. It took me a long time to understand my own. My rabbi arranged for a local rabbi to come and talk with my father, and for *Vidui*, the final letting go.

My father continued to deteriorate, and the cancer increasingly lessened his ability to think and respond. My father, who loved a good joke and who had a keen mind, became befuddled. He kept asking to go to the hospital, where he'd be made well. That abruptly stopped, and my father started to tell me that he was fine. He told me repeatedly that he had seen the doctor and the doctor had given him a "clean bill of health." I shouldn't worry about him. In a lifetime of loving me and with all the generosity of his heart, he tried to the end to protect me even from his death. When he spoke of death at all, he talked of seeing his parents again and of not being afraid. All this almost abstract view was as if he weren't talking about himself and was as close as he was able to come to his own dying.

"It's not when you're dead that you need someone to do for you," he said, "but what you do for the living that matters." It was a lesson he taught me well because he lived his life that way. I found myself having conversations with God, reminding God of my father's goodness, asking that he not suffer, and waging a battle within myself when I prayed for him. I knew that I couldn't ask either for healing or for his death and found myself asking for what was good for my father. I knew I was letting go. When he died, as much as the pain of loss engulfed me, I also believed it was best for him.

Death is inevitable, but being prepared isn't. A chance opportunity of a program at my synagogue enabled us to pro-

Caring for Our Parents
by Making Decisions Together

RABBI THOMAS A. LOUCHHEIM

Respecting Our Parents

Our world holds on so dearly to the illusion of youth that we have denied the reality and victory of growing older. So much attention is given to looking young and acting young that to grow older in our society is seen as a failure. Betty Friedan, in her preface to her book *The Fountain of Age*, recounts a recent birthday:

> When my friends threw a surprise party on my sixtieth birthday, I could have killed them all. Their toasts seemed hostile, insisting as they did that I publicly acknowledge reaching sixty, pushing me out of life, as it seemed, out of the race. Professionally, politically, personally, sexually. Distancing me from their fifty-, forty-, thirty-year-old selves. Even my own kids, though they loved me, seemed determined to be part of the torture. I was almost taunting in my response, assuring my friends that they, too, would soon be sixty if they lived that long. But I was depressed for weeks after that birthday party, felt removed from them all. I could not face being sixty.[1]

As Jews, we are taught that the elderly person is one to be respected. The Torah does not teach us how to think about the elderly, but rather prescribes how we are to act when we encounter an aged person. In

Leviticus 19:32 we learn, "You shall rise before the aged and show respect for the old [*zakein*]; you shall fear your God: I am *Adonai*." When a *zakein* enters the room, our tradition teaches us that we should rise from our seat in respect, a reminder not to disregard or ignore the presence of an elder. We are to take time out from our busy life to be patient with, to honor, and to give consideration to those older than ourselves. Regardless of scholarly achievements or whether the person is Jewish or not, we should respect the *zakein*.[2]

As our parents age, we need to consider our responsibilities toward them. It is clear from our Jewish sources that it is our responsibility to care for our parents when they need help. But what is it practically that we are able to do? During the early part of the twentieth century, the issue of filial responsibility versus government aid began to be tested. Beginning in 1935 in the Untied States, Social Security began to provide basic economic maintenance for increasing numbers of older people. Even though government and welfare agencies today assist in removing some of the financial burdens from families, children must still attend to the many other emotional and personal needs of their parents. There are critical decisions to be made, and if children and parents can sit down to have frank discussions about options and make these decisions before a crisis occurs, there will be fewer problems and conflicts in the future. Making these decisions early on and together is one of the most important ways we can show our parents respect. Even the youngest family members are affected by the events in the lives of their grandparents. Their attitudes toward the elderly will be shaped by the situations and attitudes within the family circle.

Taking care of aging parents and having to make choices that will affect their aging process are issues that will affect more and more of us each year, even as we ourselves begin to think about our own aging. Today there are 9 million Americans 80 years old and older. According to the U.S. Census Bureau, this figure will increase to 15 million in 2025, and by 2050 there will be 31 million Americans over 80, including 1 million over 100. Although there is an increasing potential for health problems as one gets older, the majority of our elderly live within their communities and require little assistance, sometimes even well into their 90's.

The following are some of the myths about the elderly:

1. *As the population ages, there will be more grumpy old men and women.* False. This is true only if they were grumpy in their thirties.
2. *Most elderly people will live in a nursing home.* False. About four out of five Americans over eighty live in the community and not in a nursing home.
3. *Elderly people are senile.* False. Only one in twenty Americans over sixty-five has dementia. Dementia is not to be confused with delirium, which is an acute state of confusion characterized by the inability to pay attention to the environment and surroundings. Its hallmark is confusion rather than memory loss. Treatment of delirium is often successful.[3]
4. *Disability is rising as our population ages.* False. As gains in the health industry are made, disabilities in those over sixty-five are actually declining.
5. *Old age is a time of idyllic serenity and tranquility, a time to just relax and enjoy the fruits of one's labors. Once you reach a certain age, you can't be productive anymore.* True and false. It depends on the individual. There are more and more individuals who continue as they age to do what they always have done. Retirement is often not a consideration. Likewise, many older individuals spend their time volunteering to help others.
6. *Elderly people are resistant to change.* False. This depends more on lifelong personality traits than on one's age.

People are shaped mostly by their own personal history, family environment, and inherent personality characteristics. A complex mix of physical, emotional, and social forces determines how one ages, and a problem in any one of these areas can upset the balance.

The aging process can be made more manageable, and there are steps to take that can add years to a person's life. For example, by scheduling regular eye examinations, a degenerative condition can be caught early and treated successfully. The four most common causes of visual impairment in people over sixty-five years are macular degeneration, cataracts, glaucoma, and diabetic retinopathy.[4] Older persons fear going blind because of the psychological isolation and physical immobilization that can result. In actuality, many older people have reasonably good sight until age ninety and beyond. Much vision loss can be avoided through early diagnosis with proper screening tests and treatment of the disability.

Another example is the growth of the home health-care industry and housing plans offering the spectrum from total independence to nursing care. Those individuals who are able to live at home are less likely to decline. If a person is able to continue to live surrounded by familiar objects, their keepsakes and photographs will provide a sense of continuity, comfort, and security and will aid the memory.

When people feel they have choices and have some control over their lives, they tend to live longer.

Therefore, we must enable our parents to make as many choices for themselves as possible, for as long as is possible. We must also encourage them to be as physically and mentally active as possible. Adults with a good education, with positive social networks, who exercise, and who maintain a proper diet are less likely to get all kinds of dementia. Maintaining a certain level of activity, be it physical, social, or intellectual, can also ward off episodes of depression. Depressed individuals die sooner than comparably ill people who aren't depressed.

Intervention

Yet even with all of this planning and care, there may still come a time when we are required to take on a parenting role for our aging parents. In a world that emphasizes youth, self-actualization, individuality, and success at all cost, there is often a conflict between the values of our religious tradition and our own ideas of how best to use available time. The Beatles put it best: "Will you still need me, will you still feed me, when I'm sixty-four?" When an elderly loved one becomes dependent upon family, what is required is a major overhaul in the priorities and orientations of the family members' lives.

A familiar passage from the Mishnah teaches us that respect for other human beings is an obligation:

> These are the commandments, the fruits of which a man
> enjoys in this life while the principal endures for him to all

eternity: honoring one's father and mother, performing deeds of loving-kindness, attending the house of study morning and evening, welcoming guests, visiting the sick. . . .

Mishnah *Pei-ah* 1:1

This passage, repeated in the daily prayer service, is the link between veneration of parents and elders and providing needed care and attention to the elderly. It is underscored by the placement of the commandment of honoring one's father and mother first, followed by general and then specific acts of compassion, and finally by study of Torah. This link between the needs of growing old and acts of kindness and compassion is found in other biblical and rabbinic sources as well.

Do not reject me in my old age; do not abandon me when my strength has left me. . . . Even in old age and hoary hairs abandon me not until I have declared Your strength unto the next generation, Your might to everyone that is to come.

Psalm 71:9, 18

We may be faced with the need to provide greater support and care to older family members. We may witness a period of functional and mental decline. Some of the symptoms may go unrecognized, be ignored, or be attributed to the normal aging process. It is important to become aware of the normal signs of aging in order to know when to ask for assistance from a physician or other health-care professional. Dr. Mark Beers has written that aging individuals and their children need to share in the task of maintaining good health, along with the health-care team, and to know how to recognize the signs of an impending medical problem.[5] Educating ourselves about potential problems and available resources is part of the obligation toward our parents spoken of in our sources.

After one has accepted that change is occurring, planning and the use of appropriate services can avert a potential crisis. Regardless of the reasons leading up to a crisis situation, when an emergency occurs, immediate steps must be taken to intervene on behalf of the older adult.

Types of Potential Crises

Crises in Activities of Daily Living (ADLs)

Crises in ADLs are the second most frequently reported crises among older adults (dementia-related crises are the first). These include changes in eating, bathing, toileting, dressing, and grooming. Frequently changes in these behaviors occur over time. Individuals will often adapt their behavior to the dysfunction.

Management of this type of crisis includes professional assessment of the individual's functional ability. Arrangements can then be made to compensate for loss in particular functions, which may range from vocational therapy to the possibility of a temporary or permanent move into a care facility.

Medical Crises

Medical crises are typically acute in nature, requiring immediate medical attention in a hospital or emergency care facility. These can involve falls, broken bones, stroke, heart attack, and drug overdose. Once the patient is stabilized, plans for the person's care need to be made after the emergency has passed.

Mental Health Crises

Mental health crises cover a wide range of behaviors, from mental illness, alcoholism, and drug abuse to family conflicts, acute emotional distress, dementia, and possible thoughts of suicide.

The reported incidents of mental health crises are much lower than for ADLs and medical crises. The reasons are that adults are unlikely to ask for help and, even when they perceive a problem, resist submitting to counseling and treatment. Referrals most often come from nurses, social workers, and family members. However, family members are often reluctant to refer their parent to a counselor or a facility out of embarrassment or in the hope that the behavior is only temporary and will pass.

Intervention can range from in-home assessment to counseling over the phone, to admission to a psychiatric treatment facility. The type of intervention depends upon the seriousness of the situation, a determination that should be made by a qualified professional.

Assessing the Situation
and Determining a Course of Action

Involving Family

The key in making any decisions is to hold a family conference that includes all members of the family. If all family members cannot be present, include people by phone or computer. If there are members of the family who cannot be accommodated at this meeting, fill them in and have a second meeting. Some families meet once a year or more frequently. The ideal is to make plans *with*, not *for*, the elderly person. The best idea is to speak to parents when they are well physically and emotionally. Explore what they would want in a given situation. It is a mistake to make plans behind a parent's back. Our tradition teaches that even "a dying person is to be considered a living being in all matters"[6]—all the more so for someone in reasonably good health.

The other good reason to have a family conference is not only for the children to understand and discuss the desires of their parents, but also to assist in sorting out solutions and tasks. The care of one's parents should not be a business-as-usual decision. Their care should be a group effort. Ideally, siblings should assist each other so that the care is not a burden on any one individual.

Gathering Information in Advance

You will need to gather information about finances, medical care options, housing, and community resources. Also, you must take into consideration the emotional responses from your parents and yourself.

Finances/Legal

In order to make realistic arrangements with your parents, you need to assess their financial status. You will need information about income, assets, insurance coverage, and the cost of keeping up your parents' current lifestyle. It is, of course, important to be sensitive in your approach to this touchy subject.

Important questions to ask your parents include the following:

1. Where are financial papers located?
2. What are the names and phone numbers of the parents' bank, accountant, and attorney?
3. Do parents have a will, and where it is located?
4. Are trust provisions up to date?
5. In the event of a crisis, who will take on fiduciary roles?
6. Do parents have powers of attorney and health-care directives (advance directives, living wills, do not resuscitate orders)?

The last item on this list is important because it needs to be decided who will act as agents if a parent becomes incapacitated. If a child is acting as the agent, then it would be a good idea to determine the parent's wishes in advance. This is also true of funeral arrangements. Where does the parent want to be buried? Is cremation being considered? Discussion of these and related issues will help reduce the tension and anxiety later on during a crisis.

Check with the Social Security Administration about benefits. Benefits become available at age sixty-five; one may also retire at sixty-two with reduced monthly benefits or at seventy-two with increased monthly benefits. Contact the Social Security Administration (800-772-1213) for more information.

Medicare is the federal government's health insurance program for people sixty-five or older, disabled persons, and others. Individuals must enroll. At this time, Medicare coverage does not include extended nursing home care, prescription drugs, custodial care, dentures and routine dental care, eyeglasses, hearing aides, and vision and hearing examinations.

There are other considerations to think about. Look into the Specified Low Income Medicare Beneficiary Program (SLMB), Medicare HMOs, Medicare Supplemental Insurance—Medigap, Long Term Care Insurance, Supplemental Security Income (SSI), and Tax Relief.

Medical Care Options
An old man goes to see his doctor complaining that his knee hurts. The doctor says, "Well, that's to be expected at your age." The old man replies, "But Doc, my other knee is just as old, and it feels fine!"

Every individual ages differently. Aging should not be considered a disease. While there is yet no way to stop or reverse the aging process, there are many things that can be done to improve and maintain a healthy lifestyle. The U.S. Department of Health and Human Services has identified five areas to enhance wellness and achieve healthy aging:

1. Practice good nutritional habits.
2. Exercise regularly.
3. Avoid excessive stress.
4. Limit alcohol and drug use.
5. Avoid smoking.

Encourage your parents to see a primary care physician on an annual basis at the very least. If the physician is not trained in geriatrics or is not experienced in treating older adults, consider consulting another qualified professional with appropriate skills. Concerned family members should ask questions and request explanations of treatment. If multiple drugs from the same or different physicians have been prescribed, consult either the primary doctor or a pharmacist about drug interactions.

Dementia is a unique area and can create great friction within a family. Contacting the Alzheimer's Association can be helpful. *Tears in God's Bottle*, by Wayne Ewing, can also be an important resource. Although not written from a Jewish perspective, it can help family members face the intense emotional and theological problems associated with this kind of illness.

A diagnosis of terminal illness is important to discuss with the whole family. This is extremely difficult for all involved, including the patient, the spouse, children, and even the doctor. The goal should be to provide as much support as possible for the terminally ill person by spending time with him or her, allowing expressions of anger and denial, respecting the person's wishes, and providing spiritual as well as emotional support. One of the finest institutions for assisting a family in dealing with terminal illness is the hospice.

Hospice care is provided at home whenever possible. Sometimes it is provided in a hospice facility or within another health-care institution. Hospice care provides support and care for terminally ill persons *and* their families in the last stages of illness, allowing a person to die with dignity. Jewish law prescribes that one may neither hasten death nor postpone death. This is the philosophy of hospice care as well.

It is never too early to educate yourself about the different medical care options available in your community, including family care, respite care, home health care, and hospice care. Being knowledgeable about available resources is part of the care that you can provide your parents.

Housing

There may be a time when parents may no longer be able to manage independently at home. Find out about alternatives in advance and, whenever possible, with your parents' input. This reduces anxiety and provides your parents with an all-important opportunity to make the decision for themselves. Some options may include full- or part-time help at home, the use of community homemaker services, living with a child or a friend, adult care homes, a continuing care retirement community (CCRC), and a nursing home.[7]

If your family needs to choose an alternative living arrangement for a parent, check the Better Business Bureau, and get references and recommendations from others. Inspect the premises for odors, cleanliness, noise levels, and call lights, and make sure that there are no evident safety issues.

Community Resources

In addition to the medical care options, it is also recommended to start as soon as possible to determine what general resources on aging are available to you and your family. All states have a service network to assist the elderly. The federal government's Administration on Aging requires each state to have a state unit on aging to implement services for the elderly. Check with a local Jewish home for the aging or Jewish Family and Children's Services. There are professionals in these organizations who can help cut through the red tape and assist in finding the resources your family needs. Some local Jewish nursing homes or community organizations offer resources like the *Handmaker Elder Care Handbook*.[8]

Emotional Concerns

We have an obligation to take care of our parents. The Talmud provides us with numerous examples, like that of Rabbi Tarfon, who would make himself into a human ladder to help his aged mother climb into bed (JT *Kiddushin* 1:7). According to Jewish law, children are obligated to respond to the physical needs of their parents. Yet their emotional well-being is important as well.

The most important thing we can do is to listen. Empathize, but don't pity. Understand, but don't condescend. There is a story told about a Reb Mosheh. After Reb Mosheh's death, a friend said of him: "If there had been someone to whom he could have talked, he would still be alive."[9] If you are bothered by the fact that your parent or grandparent seems to always talk about the same old stuff, the real mitzvah of *g'milut chesed* (loving-kindness) would be to listen for a change. As we learn from *Sefer Hachinuch*, a thirteenth-century text, the *z'keinim*, our "elders," have a lifetime of wisdom to teach us. Ask about their childhood. Find out what it was like growing up Jewish in their hometown. Ask what legacy they want to leave in the business world. What value do they want to pass on to their children and grandchildren? Suggest that they write letters or ethical wills to their children and grandchildren.[10]

As important as the practical help we can offer are the consideration and the sensitivity to the changes that occur when family members age. Not only are they going through changes that require them to make adjustments in their lifestyles; we too must make adjustments in ours. Special care needs to be taken to ensure that the stresses on each individual and the family unit are not overwhelming. Be attentive to emotional responses resulting in adjustments to the family's day-to-day routine. How each family rallies around a crisis is different. Every member will behave differently. Be attentive to signs of anger, grief, fear, denial, and guilt. Attempt to make adjustments, being sensitive to a parent's needs and the needs of different members of the family.

While we must make sure to take care of the emotional needs of our parents, we cannot be good caregivers if we neglect our own emotional needs. Caregiving is emotionally and physically stressful. You must deal with a parent's state of mind and body as well as your own. Recognize physical signs of stress—hypertension, headaches, and chest and abdominal pain. There may be psychological stress symptoms—fatigue, insomnia, depression, loss of appetite, and irritability. Here are some guidelines for taking care of yourself, the caregiver:[11]

1. Set limits. Know where to draw the line. At the same time, emphasize what the caregiver can be counted on to do.
2. Refrain from taking on any of a parent's responsibilities before it becomes necessary. This undermines your parent's self-esteem and autonomy.
3. Join a support group. It can be helpful to share experiences with others in similar circumstances.
4. Share as much of the caregiving as possible, with siblings, relatives, friends, and even members of a congregation. If a family member doesn't want to share in the caregiving, give him or her specific tasks to do.
5. Make time for rest, good nutrition, exercise, and maintaining your own social connections, all of which will serve to revitalize and recharge you and make you a better caregiver.

Working with Our Parents to Meet Their Needs

The key to caring for the elderly is to remember that everyone has emotional, spiritual, physical, and intellectual needs. Be sure that you can attend to as much of them as you are able. This provides the individual with a greater quality of life, not just length of days.[12]

When I first became a rabbi, I entered a nursing home in Kansas City to visit my first resident there. I no sooner walked in the door when she cried out, "I just want to die. My children put me in this place to die." We spent an hour talking about her now-deceased husband, her life, and her children. When I left the room, she was looking forward to my next visit. If we can attend to some of the needs and desires of our aging parents, maybe they won't feel discarded. Maybe we just need to learn how to listen better.

If parents are resistant to your suggestions, be ready to suggest options. Give them time to think about proposed solutions. If the situation needs an immediate solution, stress how important their safety and welfare are to you. Your parents may not listen to you, but they may listen to the sage advice of others. Enlist the aid of a family friend, the primary physician, your rabbi, or your parents' rabbi. Find out how your synagogue's members might be able to help your family. The key is to respond to your parents' needs. Listen to their voice, not your own inner voice.

Just because someone is aging does not mean that creativity, curiosity, and spontaneity become dormant. Cervantes, Voltaire, Goethe, Tolstoy, Picasso, and Grandma Moses all started or bloomed late in life. Encourage expression in areas of interest. There are many classes available to seniors at local community colleges, parks, and recreation centers, which may spark an interest.

As a person ages, there is often a greater appreciation for the life cycle. Individuals may gain a personal sense of their own life cycle. They may develop a greater interest in religion, philosophy, or art. If so, try to accommodate this recognition with ritual or appropriate events or ceremonies.

The aging person may have a sense of consummation or fulfillment in life. Serenity and wisdom are often derived from resolution of personal conflicts and a review of life. Material success is not necessary. Having survived great odds is to have succeeded. As Rabbi Alvin Fine wrote, "Victory lies not at some high point along the way, but in having made the journey stage by stage."

Nachman of Bratzlav said, "Old men bring stability to Israel and give good counsel to the people. The prosperity of a country is in accordance with its treatment of the aged."[13] Old age is not a disease. It is a part of life. If we focus simply on symptoms of aging, we are not giving our elders the best care possible. We must meet their social, spiritual, and intellectual needs as well.

While it is wonderful to be able to be financially generous with your parents, not everyone is able to offer that kind of support. But all of us must make the effort to help fulfill their emotional and spiritual needs. This is truly the fulfillment of the mitzvah "Honor your father and mother."

Growing Old Isn't for the Faint of Heart: Making Decisions Together

෮ ෯

Rabbi Jonathan P. Kendall

My mother's hair is white and exceedingly fine. About once a month, I take her to the beauty parlor. The man who does her hair is a Japanese fellow who dresses like a ninja and cuts very quickly, with almost blinding speed. I always observe this samurai ritual from afar, watching as her hair falls like gossamer snow around the chair. Haiku and other snippets of thought and little particles of keepsakes from other times fly around the room. Finally, a circle of white forms around her feet in delicate drifts, and it is time to go. How many years and how many trips to the beauty parlor has she been able to number? For a fleeting moment, I think about my own outings as a child for haircuts. My mother stood apart and watched, encouraging me, smiling, buoying my spirits, standing in the place I am now. I hated haircuts and the barber. It was a traumatic experience until I was at least seven or eight or maybe even nine. Now our chairs, our positions, have been reversed. Now, it is I who stands and smiles and encourages.

With some kind of alchemy to which only those of us who have "lived through it" can attest, the parent becomes the child and the child becomes the parent. This may be the most uneven and unsettling part of life's journey. In the end, it wasn't any day of reckoning or any one cataclysmic event that brought us to this juncture. My mother's decline was glacial, organic, and practically imperceptible. Over the course of a year, she went from being a cautiously mobile Mom to being a wheelchair-bound Mother. There were other intimations of her physical descent. She felt totally secure being alone in my home—or so she said—but I saw that posture as bravado, a combination of denial and the Jewish mother's mantra of "I don't want to be a burden . . ." As a consequence, I was nervous whenever I ventured from the house. An evening out occasioned calls home; a weekend away became a major production; a vacation for any length of time required planning worthy of a military campaign. And even as I write those words, a wave of shame washes over me. Was it my inconvenience or the time I had to devote to her care that forced the issue? I hope not. Is this what the Torah means by honoring parents or rising up to show deference to the aged? Sometimes, especially in the highly charged, emotional world of children with aging parents, a knowledge of tradition and text can work against us and not for us.

First, the great cruelty, the rotten divine joke: with infinite wisdom, genetic hard-wiring and modern medicine, the Lord of All Worlds gave my mother more years than many. A college graduate who worked her entire life because she was never content to be "just a housewife," my mother was the poster girl for frenetic, vital, purposeful activity. Though degreed in fine art, during World War II she busied herself with the Red Cross as a case worker. From there, she graduated to doing medical social work for the Easter Seal Society and finally stopped her daily toils as the executive director of a charitable trust at the age of 71.

Self-sufficient, self-reliant, creative, inventive, social, and deeply committed to synagogue and community, the only thing keeping her "down" was a deteriorating body. Her mind remains as sharp, as analytical, as gifted as it always has been. That is a blessing, but one that is mixed.

Two years ago it became clear, at least to me, that she required "assisted living." The very phrase has a discordant sound and unpleasant implications. The simple acts that we take for granted—rising from our beds, preparing our meals, shopping for food and clothing, bathing—the litany of everyday life—all of a sudden require assistance. After driving becomes an impossibility—another wrenching assault on independence—our entire view of the world is altered. If the car is a symbol of autonomy, then what of the simpler and more basic elements of living for which one now requires "assistance"? These were among the kaleidoscopic thoughts that kept brushing against my conscience as I watched my mother's hair float to the ground. And I kept hearing—again and again—an accusation: how can I abandon her when she never abandoned me? And is a placement in an assisted living facility tantamount to desertion? Truth be told, the beauty parlor became a source of enormous anxiety for me. Was it the fact that she was no longer beautiful—at least youthfully so—that this woman who once carried herself so elegantly and proudly now needed help to leave her wheelchair? Was this ritual of personal aesthetics a metaphor that captured the harsh juxtaposition of parent and child?

As a rabbi, I have watched in dismay as parents become more and more feeble and slight. Inevitably, one of them dies and the survivor—unable to fend for themselves—lands in a nursing home or assisted living facility while children and grandchildren are still "up north" or "out west" or someplace else far removed. I have listened to every convoluted rationale and excuse for these placements and never understood them. It was as if the distance somehow neutralized the impact of the decision. Out of sight, out of mind. Perhaps my deep-seated distaste for families who "warehouse" their parents and grandparents kept me from making any decision for so very long. There was a kind of paralysis that hovered over the entire issue. I was uncharacteristically indecisive and terribly conflicted. And my own childhood and adolescence played a role in my ambivalence.

My grandmother, rest her dear soul, had lived with us for the final eight years of her life. We provided the "assisted living." No one contemplated a facility of any sort. Her presence in the house may have cramped my style during those teenage years of mine, but any alternative was unthinkable. My memories of Grandma are not filled with any kind of resentment. They are as tender as can be. A piece of that sweetness is the knowledge that we did everything we could to make her last years gentle, humane, and brimming with care. No guilt there, to be sure. When I changed pulpits seven years ago, Mom was already living in a "retirement community." There was no doubt in my mind or my heart that I would take her with me. I would not be one of those children who left a parent alone. By my lights, an only child had no other option.

But that was then, and this is now.

Now comes the moment of truth. There are many scripts we write in an effort to put our best foot forward, to convince the other party of our sincerity and the wisdom of our decisions. Every facet of life is filled with this scripting mechanism. Part of that is, undeniably, to convince ourselves. These affirmations are neatly packaged and wrapped graciously in logic and reason. The anxiety that rose in my gorge before "the presentation" was as powerful as any I can remember. I fully expected that there would be protestations and challenges, but in the end, all of the concerns were for naught. Mom agreed that it was, indeed, time.

At that moment, I made a terrible error in judgment. I took her with me to visit various assisted living facilities. If I had this to do over again, I would have gone alone and found the "right one" first. I live in a small community, and the number of these institutions is not extensive. Some are beautiful and far beyond her means and mine. Others are abysmal, depressing places filled with unconscionable human desolation. We visited one—very popular, I might add—and the excursion into the lobby was enough to kill the deal. At least thirty residents were lined up in a semicircle of wheelchairs. Some spoke to each other, others conversed with the disembodied spirits of long-lost family and friends; most slept, and one— I was sure—had expired. It was a geriatric tableau of hell. We never made it to the reception desk for our grand tour.

After fits and starts, we did find an assisted living facility that was quite lovely. The accommodations were capacious, the public rooms were well maintained, they permitted small pets (which meant that the cat could go with her, an essential selling point), and the residents were reasonably homogeneous in terms of education and life experience.

And so began the preparations for "the move." "I never thought that I would be moving again . . . " was the refrain I heard most often. It was never said in a mean-spirited or accusatory way; I just allowed myself to hear it in those terms. In the end, I was far more agitated about this relocation than was my mother. If there were "abandonment issues" swirling in the air, they were all mine. None of the rationalizations I brought to the table seemed to neutralize them. I just felt rotten about this turn of events; there is no other way to describe it.

The morning we moved in was bright and sunny. I'm looking at that last phrase, and I am struck by the choice of language. I didn't write (or think) "the morning SHE moved." I thought and felt that "we" were moving. A piece of me was going with her. A strange combination of regret and relief greeted me on that day. The regrets were about my own inadequacies: not being able to care for her as I believed a son should, not "living up to my end of the bargain" in this dance of parents-and-children, knowing that time was not on her side and that this move would mean a separation that presaged the longer separation to come. The relief factor was a little less compelling, but it did assert itself. There was comfort in knowing that someone would be "looking in" on Mom regularly, that she would have help with the things she needed and a community in which she could live that might mitigate some of the isolation she was beginning to feel living with me.

The "old folks home" (as she calls it) sits on a hill adjacent to the Intracoastal Waterway. It is a pretty site and really quite majestic in appearance. Her apartment is on the second floor overlooking a courtyard but close enough to the elevator to insure easy ingress and egress. The move complete, the cat ensconced, the furniture and pictures arranged, the cable hooked up, the phones tested—and now it was time to go. As I walked down the hall to the elevator, I was seized by a feeling of déjà vu. When finally my kids had been unpacked and installed in their dorms and were pushing me out the door, I had felt as though a signal, watershed moment had been reached in their lives and mine. They would no longer be under my roof and everyday fixtures in my life. At best, now they would be visitors. Still connected by the umbilical cord of unconditional love and devotion, they were now in a different category of human existence as they related to me. This was a natural progression. The fledglings do leave the nest. They are supposed to do that. How ironic that the same feelings of loss and transformation should accompany this leave-taking.

Just as people advised me to "drop" the kids and beat a hasty retreat, so they counseled the same here, to allow Mom to adjust to her new environment without any intrusiveness that might somehow inhibit the process of adjustment. It wasn't easy.

"How was dinner?" I asked later that night on the phone. My mother never complained about food, and she wasn't going to begin now. But her tablemates were another story. One thing I have learned in this transaction of placing parents in assisted living or nursing facilities is that you would do well to make sure that every "t" is crossed and every "i" is dotted. The three people with whom she ate dinner were in varying stages of mental decline. One, she reported, only asked her name "at least fifty times."

"Go to the director and let her know that you absolutely must be seated at a table with folks who are 'with it,'" I said.

My mother is no shrinking violet. This she did, and for a time her new tablemates became important pieces of her adjustment. Two were professional women and one, a lovely Dutch gentleman who had suffered a stroke, made meals and communal events within the institution bearable and even quite pleasant.

The variety of people in assisted living institutions covers all the bases. There are some who are completely sentient.

Their problems are mobility related. There are others who look as though they could run a respectable marathon but have no idea who or where they are. The train that runs between these two poles is a local; it makes stops at every point between full faculties and galloping senility. For those who enter an assisted living center with their wits completely about them, their encounters with people whose awareness has fallen on hard and irretrievable times can be depressing and jarring. This is why I say that my mother's mental state is a mixed blessing.

The predicament of dining companions solved, then came the issue of time.

The physicist Stephen Hawking has written some remarkable books on the subject of time. In the far reaches of the universe, it is compressible. We know from our own observations that in our childhood, time appears to move very slowly. As we grow older, it seems to move with inexorable speed. Here's a newsflash for Dr. Hawking: if you are in assisted living or in a nursing home, time slows down again. It barely moves at all, and instead of telescoping, it becomes a vessel of listlessness and resignation. Hours, days, and weeks collide with each other in a jumble of desultory monotony. There is often an aimless and indiscriminate current of time interrupted by diversions that in the world outside, the world "before," would never have captured our interest. At eighty-six, my mother has never played bingo. She should begin now? And five times a week, no less?

I have many friends who teach at the university level. They are brilliant, mature, and gifted people—except when they speak of the "administration." At that point, they become teenagers, filled with resentment and often snickering grievances against what becomes the surrogate parent:

the dean, the provost, the department chair. Life in institutions for the aged is pretty much the same. There, the "enemy" is the "management." They are the ones responsible for the less-than-three-star cuisine, the periodic surliness of the staff, and the quality of the entertainment and activities. There was no way on God's green earth that my mother was going to tolerate a fellow with an accordion and a harmonica as any credible representation of "culture." She was and is a painter, and she convinced the "management" to open an art studio. She even volunteered to give lessons. And so began her real salvation in assisted living. Her "class" has come and gone, but her paintings now grace the lobby, and the "management" uses the studio as a selling point to prospective residents. She has become a corporate asset, and likely future residents and their families are brought to her—not only because she is coherent, but also because she fills her days with more than just ennui.

In some ways, both my mother and I are fortunate in this situation, in spite of the emotional hardships. The assisted living facility is two miles from my house. I can "drop in" at almost any time (feeling better when I visit, worse when I leave). She still volunteers one morning per week at the temple, answering the telephones, stuffing envelopes, and mailing fliers. Two younger women in the congregation paint with her on a weekly basis in "her" studio, and a group of older congregants come for lunch once or twice a month. All of this creates considerable and understandable envy among those residents who have only the establishment and themselves, their four walls and their televisions with which to occupy their days. A supportive community is an indispensable ingredient in this odyssey. Without the additional leavening of a life "outside the walls," even the most luxurious and sumptuous of placements becomes nothing more than an institution. The resident can evolve into an inmate in a very short period of time. The psychological and physical tolls are palpable. Unless children and the community are willing to work hard together to insure that those conditions are not the norm, we take the golden years and tarnish them most cruelly. The damage done by neglect and indifference is devastating.

For the past ten years a variety of physical ailments has conspired to make my mother's life less than complete and often quite discomfiting. As a result, I have come to envy those who are able to negotiate their days with a minimum of *tzuris* and close them peacefully, gathered beneath God's wings with a gentle kiss. Then there are those for whom the last years are a struggle and an ordeal. We leave it to the physicians to neutralize the pain. It falls to us to retaliate against the isolation, the emotional upheavals, the loss of self and self-respect, the surrender of independence—all of the affective tribulations to which our parents are subjected. It is a terrible burden they carry only when it is borne alone.

In the foyer by the elevators on the first floor there is a baby-grand player piano. It is almost always going—some generic Scott Joplin loop that plays on and on. As I come and go, there is one resident—an old woman—who sits attentively, foot tapping, head swaying, syncopated rhythm from dawn to dusk. There is no honor in this, no respect, no tenderness or sensitivity. There is no companionship, no camaraderie, no rapport. She is very much alone. I look at her as I pass, and I see only despair. But then, I wonder, is the despair mine or hers? And is that despair more about her or more about me? Is it more about yesterday or more about tomor-

Jewish Values and Sociopsychological Perspectives on Aging

DR. ROBERT L. KATZ, Z"l

Despite vast medical progress we know relatively little about the phenomenon of aging. The term itself is imprecise and ambiguous. We do know some things about the processes of aging, one of these being that we begin to "age" while we are still in our teens. We age at different rates; aging has different meanings for different people; to be aged may be a chronological variable because Picasso at ninety-plus had more vigor than some of us who would be loosely categorized as being of "middle age." Medical researchers only recently discovered that the arteries of young men can be "aged," while some people attain a "ripe old age" with cardiovascular systems resembling those associated with much younger people. Are we "aged" if we choose to retire at the age of forty-five or fifty, or are we "aged" when we first become eligible for Social Security? Do we become "aged" when we leave our own apartment and move into a residence complex where our fellow residents are classified as being "elderly?" There simply is no unequivocal meaning for the "aging" or "aged"; moreover, we cannot be sure when we are speaking in the language of physiology, psychology, economic status, athletic ability and physical coordination, medicine and health status, political influence, familial role, or something else.

More than most of us realize, aging is a state of mind; we are what *we* think we are, the ways we perceive ourselves, and the ways we imagine

Reprinted, with changes, from *Pastoral Psychology* 24, no. 229 (winter 1975): 135–150.

our family and our community to perceive us. Aging is, at the very least, a relative term. A famous symphony conductor, now in his nineties, is still at work and now plans to build a new home in Venice. According to the calendar, he is indeed "old." But by what scientific, "objective" standards shall Leopold Stokowski be called old? If we speak of a so-called "life-span," he has comfortably exceeded the threescore and ten years of life cited in Psalm 90 but has some years to go before attaining the 120 years that Deuteronomy asserts Moses achieved. We conclude, then, that "aging" is an arbitrary nomenclature, a variable, subject to the widest interpretation. It is, therefore, important to consider the inputs both of religion and of science in trying to expand our grasp of the phenomenon of aging in our culture and in reaching for a system of values or attitudes that will be intelligent, realistic, and spiritually valid. Our statement will consider a number of variables, among them a variety of attitudes explicit and implicit in the tradition of Judaism.

Aging in Jewish Literature

According to one of the rabbinic homilies on the Bible, in early times it was not ordinarily the custom to take note of distinctions in age, even between father and son. When the distinction was introduced, it was for reasons of resolving an issue of status. Such was the case of Abraham and Isaac, according to the Rabbis.[1]

> Until Abraham's time the young and the old were not distinguished from each other; consequently young people would jest with Abraham, taking him for their companion, whereas the old addressed Isaac in a manner becoming a man of years. This induced Abraham to pray to God for an outward token of dignity and honor for those advanced in years and the Lord, granting his wish, said, "Thou shalt be the first upon whose head the silver crown of old age shall rest."[2]

Aging here, as in so many Jewish sources, is presented as a valued status, one with privileges denied to others. Another source holds that old age is in itself not necessarily honorable. A man can be venerable without being old, while others live long without achieving character. For the Rabbis, the ideal state was to attain both old age and honor.

Well known are the statements in the Bible mandating respect for the aged. In Leviticus 19:32, we read "Thou shalt rise up before the hoary head and honor the face of the old man." According to Proverbs 16:31, "the hoary head is a crown of glory." Wisdom is associated with the experience of being old, as in Job 12:12, "Wisdom is with the aged, and understanding is the length of days." At the same time, doubt is expressed about the inevitable accretion of wisdom with age. In Psalm 119:10, the poet claims that he is wiser than the aged because he has excelled them in piety. In the Mishnah, a post biblical work (in Ethics of the Fathers), note is taken of the fact that a new jar can be full of old wine (wisdom) and an old one may not even contain new wine (*Pirkei Avot* 4:20), but elsewhere in the context we are informed that learning from the aged is like drinking old wine. A talmudic source goes so far as to maintain that the older scholars grow, the greater their wisdom becomes (an opinion possibly reflecting the age of the speaker).

Historically speaking, the Jewish community has tended to demonstrate a care for the aged that is often taken to be exemplary. The esteem in which the aged were held was expressed in tangible form by a pattern of institutions caring for their needs. Even to this day, Jews devote considerable time, energy, and resources to providing for the aged so that Jewish solicitude is almost a stereotype. In the solidarity of the Jewish family, as it evolved almost to the present, we may find an explanation for this care. Each member of the community felt responsible for the other and the aged were notably honored. In the Jewish religious system, elders who interpreted the Torah, who transmitted it to successive generations, and who, in terms of family structure and in the value-set of Judaism, commanded a loving authority and respect. Jewish community life had an integrity of its own, even as Jewish cultural and religious life maintained its continuity, adapting to a changing environment and yet retaining the "chain of tradition." In the Riesman typology of the personality types, the tradition-directed, as contrasted with the inner- and other-directed, could be taken as a paradigm for the role of the mature, if not the aged, in the Jewish family system.[3] Since they were the custodians of the tradition, they occupied a preferred status. However, this reverence for the aged is not as intact or as consistent in contemporary society. The Jewish family has accommodated to rapid social change and has assimilated many values typical of the other-directed society. The solidarity of the Jewish family today, while still remarkable, is beginning to exhibit some signs of fragmentation. Only recently investigators have found numbers of the Jewish aged abandoned and ignored in pockets of poverty in cities like New York and Miami. Sociological investigation indicates that some prevailing conceptions of Jewish family life must be updated and revised. But Jewish concern for the aged can, even today, hardly be dismissed as a stereotype. A deeply ingrained commitment continues to make this concern distinctive in a society that is conspicuously youth-oriented and that is directed by a peer culture largely cut loose from the past and from older, more stable patterns of family organization.

The Stages of Life

Since one of the tasks of this essay is to examine values and perspectives in Judaism rather than to review specific programs for the aged, we have been dealing primarily with religious literature. In general, we find a convergence between values found there and in the most enlightened secular writers today in the sociopsychological sciences. But before turning to some contemporary social thinkers, we need to take note of views in Jewish tradition of the aged and their place in the life cycle. While it is not at all certain what is meant precisely by the term "aged," most cultures, including the Jewish, conceptualize the stages of life. There is a sense of change of status as an individual ages chronologically; each stage has particular functions appropriate to the individual as he moves from one to the other. While the values respecting each stage have remained largely unchanged, there has been an awareness of change in the appropriateness of certain roles and responsibilities. One of the more familiar models in modern social science is of course the Eight Stages of Man as conceptualized by Erik H. Erikson, a psychoanalyst.[4] Robert J. Havighurst, an educator, has also written of the "Developmental Task."[5] Such formulations were anticipated in Shakespeare and even earlier in the Bible and in rabbinic literature. The earliest reference to the Seven Ages of Man is by Hippocrates (357 B.C.E.).

The periodicity of human careers is most typically observed in the

Book of Ecclesiastes: "for everything there is a season and a time for every matter under heaven, a time to be born and a time to die" (3:1). There is a painfully vivid description of the phenomenon of senility in the twelfth chapter. The later years consist of "evil days" when the weak and the infirm have no pleasure in living. The images are dismal, evoking as they do the fragile and futile quality of those whose bodies are in acute decline. Nothing written since surpasses these few verses reflecting the physical deterioration of the senile. It is interesting that Maimonides, preeminent Jewish philosopher of the Middle Ages, claimed that by following a proper hygiene, a set of morals, and a diet, no one need fall ill, and one can "achieve old age needing no doctor and enjoy perfect, uninterrupted health."[6] Ecclesiastes' description is still obviously pertinent because, even allowing for the successful achievement of old age, individuals, aging as they do at individual rates, ultimately will experience some fatal infirmity of body, though not necessarily the complete list so meticulously catalogued in the Bible.

In Judaism the most familiar description of the stages of life is found in the Mishnah, Ethics of the Fathers:

> At five years old (one is fit) for the Scripture, at ten years for the Mishnah, at thirteen for (the fulfilling of) the commandments, at fifteen for the Talmud, at eighteen for the bride-chamber, at twenty for pursuing (a calling), at thirty for authority, at forty for discernment, at fifty for counsel, at sixty to be an elder, at seventy for gray hairs, at eighty for special strength, at ninety for bowed back, and at a hundred a man is as one that has (already) passed away and ceased from the world.[7]

References to the Seven Ages of Man abound in postbiblical and rabbinic literature. One source holds that a man grown old is like an ape—if he is an ignoramus, that is. But if he is a learned man, he, like David, is a king. Another source describes man regressing into a pitiable state and becoming terrorized by his imminent death. Ultimately the angel of death approaches him and asks him,

> "Dost thou recognize me?" to which he replies, "Indeed, I do; but wherefore dost thou come to me just this day?" "In order

to take thee out this world," says the angel, "for thy time has come to depart hence!" Immediately he commences to weep; and his cry pierces the world from one end to the other; addressing the angel, he exclaims, "Hast thou not already caused me to quit two worlds, to enter this world?" to which the angel finally replies: "And have I not already told thee, that against thy will thou art created, against thy will thou art born, against thy will thou livest, and against thy will thou must render account for thy actions before the Supreme King of Kings, blessed be He?"[8]

Man resists his destiny; life and death are thrust upon him, but there is something for which he is responsible. He must defend his lifestyle, to use an overworked but still useful phrase, before God. That calls for some initiative and even creativity on the part of man. At this point the reader will associate along with me the words of Erik Erikson, which resonate with the spirit of this image out of Jewish tradition, even though the Eriksonian perspective is anything but authoritarian or theological. In the Eighth Stage, Ego Integrity vs. Despair, the mature man, who works through to possess integrity, knows that he must "defend the dignity of his own life . . . for him all human integrity stands or falls with the one style of integrity of which he partakes."[9] These references to the stages of life and the age-appropriate life tasks of man also suggest the concept of the monomyth, as developed by Joseph Campbell in his study of mystic themes entitled *The Hero with a Thousand Faces*.[10] Campbell interprets the life cycle of man in the form of a "monomyth," which he feels can be identified in major mythologies. The career of man involves three phases: Separation, Initiation, and Return. The mature or aging would fulfill the function of teaching and maintain the continuity of man's traditions, after having achieved his own maturation and rediscovered the basic wisdom of the human race. Every man, in Campbell's formulation, must accomplish the odyssey of the hero. He writes, "A hero ventures forth from the world of the common day into a region of supernatural wonder: fabulous forces are here encountered and a decisive victory is won: the hero comes back from this mysterious adventure with the power to bestow boons on his fellow man.[11]

The Generations: Respect or Conflict

A recurring theme in all cultures is the accommodation of the generations to each other. Conflicts over power and privilege as between the young and the old were as overt in classic times as they are now, except that the alignment of forces has radically changed. Our society sees the aging as besieged by the young, now fighting a defensive battle. The so-called "middle-aged" (like "aging," an ambiguous term), while still in power, feel threatened by a youth-oriented society and typically attempt to identify with the young and with their images of what is humanly significant and precious.

We can better appreciate earlier vignettes of the war of the generations if we take note of some contemporary descriptions of the conflict. President John R. Silber of Boston University, who wrote so insightfully about this issue in the *Center Magazine*, makes the association himself when he mentions the Fifth Commandment.[12] If mothers and fathers had been consistently honored, it would not have been necessary for Moses to set down the commandment, "Honor your father and your mother." Silber articulated the need of each age group for the other and noted that when age groups are pitted against each other, "we are murderous gangs—one intent on filicide, the other on parricide."[13] He outlines his paradigm of the partnership of youth and age in these words:

> If we reorder time to celebrate youth and age and the gradual metamorphosis from one to the other, if we regain our sense of time and value the present differences in the recognition that each of us plays all the parts in sequence, we shall see that there is no salvation for the young or the old at the expense of either.[14]

This thought is echoed in the statement by the psychiatrist, Seymour L. Halleck, who commented that:

> A society which does not provide sufficient gratifications for the elderly will be an unhappy society for the young as well as the old. If the old are not satisfied, nobody can accept the prospects of age with equanimity . . . for any society which

cannot treat its elderly members decently is doomed to unremitting despair and chaos.[15]

Not the least critical element in the war of the generations is the raw competition for power and status. The elders, as Sebastian de Grazia wrote, never seem to die when young people wait and watch for their turn.[16] The Oedipus complex about which Freud has enlightened some three generations in this century distills the essence of generational conflict; even if the power and authority of the father in our culture are declining, Freud's paradigm is still useful in underscoring the recurring theme of competition, guilt, and hostility which reflect intrapsychic, interpersonal, and sociostructural variables.

References to social theorists would not be complete without including Margaret Mead, who discusses the generational encounter in her book *Culture and Commitment*.[17] She notes that social and technological change make the wisdom of the elders little more than items of quaint archaeological interest. In the traditional cultures, the elder could invoke his own youth to understand the world of his children. Mead asserts that the generational gap in our culture is so firmly established that no communication would be possible on that basis. The prospects are not entirely desolate, however. The septuagenarian anthropologist allows a certain amount of space for the encounter of the young and the old. Where can they meet? In the joint enterprise, writes Dr. Mead, "The children, the young, must ask the questions we would never think to ask, but enough trust must be reestablished so that the elders will be permitted to work with them on the answers." Note the word "permitted." But age still has its validity: "father is still the man who has the skill and the strength to cut down the tree to build a different kind of house." And adults are still needed as models: "We must create new models for adults who can teach their children not what to learn, but how to learn and not what they should be committed to, but the value of commitment."[18] It is because there are no guides—not just that the parents are no longer guides—that makes it necessary for young and old to find their way in an uncharted land.

The generational conflict echoes in Judaism long after the proclamation of the Fifth Commandment. The sources identify the struggle and, at the same time, hold out the prospect of a magnificent reconciliation.

Although our present conceptual apparatus is infinitely more sophisticated and our grasp of social processes is documented scientifically rather than theologically or poetically, we can still find enlightenment in the truths about man and society evident in biblical times. Familiar to many is the statement of the Psalmist (71:9) in which the venerable writer calls out to his children: "Do not throw me away in the time of old age, when my strength is failing me, do not forsake me." The resolution of the generational conflict is an irreducible requirement for man's salvation in history; without it chaos is inevitable. In Malachi we read, "Behold I will send you Elijah the prophet before the great and terrible day of *Adonai* comes. And he will turn the hearts of fathers to their children and the hearts of children to their fathers, lest I come and smite the land with a curse" 3:23–24.

It is interesting to note, *en passant*, that the impact of this historic passage is greatly diminished as reproduced in abbreviated form in the Union Prayerbook (Reform) at the climactic conclusion of the Day of Atonement services. Reference to the "great and terrible day of *Adonai*" is deleted, leaving only the soft-spoken invitation to the generations to turn to each other in love and become reconciled. The potentialities for explosive conflict are seen dimly, if at all in the prayers of reasonable and temperate moderns. But the potentialities nevertheless exist. The resentments of the Grey Panthers come to mind. The violence and repercussion of Kent State are most suggestive of Malachi. The Talmud picks up this prophetic theme in discussing the portentous pre-messianic days. "A sign of troubled times preceding the coming of the Messiah will be lack of courtesy and respect shown by the young toward their elders."[19]

The following comment on a possibly historical episode reflects the struggle for status between the young and the old. In this case, the tradition puts the young down abruptly and absolutely.

> In the days of Hadrian, when enthusiastic young men advised the rebuilding of the Temple in Jerusalem, some wise men reminded them of the event that occurred in Rehoboam's time and said, "If young people advise you to build the Temple and old men say destroy it, give ear to the latter; for the building of the young (done by) is destruction and the tearing down of the old (done by) is construction."[20]

Two visions of generational reconciliation need to be mentioned at this point, before turning to another theme. One is from the prophet Zechariah (8:4–5). It evokes the image not of violence in the street but of enchanting peace and beautiful symmetry of relationships. "Old men and women shall again sit in the streets of Jerusalem, each with staff in hand for every age. And the streets of the city shall be full of boys and girls playing in the streets." The following passage from Joel (3:1) seems congenial with the recommendation made by Margaret Mead, John R. Silber, and others that the generations form an effective partnership. The language of Joel is poetic and deeply moving.

> *And it shall come to pass afterward,*
> *that I will pour out My spirit on all flesh;*
> *your sons and your daughters shall prophesy*
> *your old men shall dream dreams,*
> *and your young men shall see visions.*

Aging and Social Class

We shall shortly consider the place of the aging in the classical theology of Judaism and note, in particular, the utopian, messianic conception of the role of the aged.

Before that discussion, however, it will be useful to review some of the value orientations of American culture vis-à-vis the aging. What part do the aging have in a culture that still follows a Protestant work ethic, adheres to a philosophy of scarcity, submits to a life style of consumerism, and still esteems individual worth in terms of productivity, achievement, and upward social mobility? Moreover, what part do the aging have in a "temporary society," which has little regard for history and tradition and which is primed for rapid technological and social change? Even leisure time activity is something that is organized, managed, and carried out on schedule. The sense of stress is pervasive; the feeling of restless striving and incessant mobility is almost inescapable. What are the prospects for those who, like it or not, do have leisure, who may or may not be "productive," and who may not fit in with a consumer-oriented society? The temporary quality of life is especially uncongenial to those whose inclination for continued accommodation and change is no longer as strong.

It is important to recognize that one of the most important variables in the phenomenon of aging is class status. We can easily become entrapped in the constraints of a middle-class orientation and find ourselves generalizing on the basis of the social group with which we are most familiar. This is typically a middle-class nation; even "lower" classes have a middle-class value system and internalize the perceptions of those normally considered more successful. When, for example, we speak of "disengagement" from the work force or use the term "role exit" (coined by Dr. Zena Smith Blau), we are really thinking of middle-class people who radically change their life style when they attain the age of retirement. They now feel called upon to restructure their lives and redefine their relationships.

These changes do not inhere in the reality of their chronological age; they are functions of a changing socioeconomic position. Upper-class members whose income has been derived from ownership of property or of stocks and bonds do not make a "role exit" when they reach sixty-two, sixty-five, or seventy. They are not vulnerable to many of the deprivations and dislocations of the middle-class aged. For the rich, the advance of the years also has significance of course, as it calls for accommodation to changes in the body and the loss of a sense of physical well-being. But there is no less self-esteem. They are not rejected by a social order that defers to power, wealth, and acknowledged social status. Far from being abandoned by their family, their friends, and the community, they continue to command respect, hold positions of leadership on boards of institutions, and maintain the quality of their life. Wealth does not command immortality, to be sure, but it normally discourages disrespect. So many of the penalties age inflicts must therefore be viewed as deprivations of social status rather than the absolute and irrevocable consequences of growing old. Children and grandchildren of the powerful rich continue to defer to them. They pay visits to the patriarch and matriarch in their winter and their summer homes. When such parents attain advanced age and require nursing care, they are not likely to be consigned to the warehouses for the aged and the infirm as is the fate of the dependent and aged poor. They will not live out their years in nursing homes, visited only occasionally and guiltily by their economically sufficient children. They do not live in fear of the erosion of their pensions and Social Security income. They know their children will not set them adrift on an ice floe. The young, in fact, are dependent on the patriarchs who still control the family fortunes.

The linkage of aging and social class cannot be emphasized too strongly. Those of us who come from middle-class backgrounds wish to excel our parents and rise above the status they have achieved. Our parents encouraged us to move upward and beyond them. They take vicarious satisfaction in our achievements and take comfort during their retirement years that they have successful children who have "made" it. This satisfaction is an antidote to the pains and deprivations of their own diminished status. In the case of the rich and the privileged, elderly parents continue to be the models to be emulated; children are content to follow in their footsteps. The aged continue to symbolize success, and their patronage is sought by community leaders, artists, and celebrities. Not for them is the state of near-panic of the man who faces retirement and the sudden reduction of income and loss of face. Most middle-aged people are unprepared for the transition into rolelessness. Their life style is to be linked to an uncertain income. But if you belong to a family of established wealth, you do not pass from one role to rolelessness with the elapse of time. You continue to practice conspicuous consumption because you have the means and you know that you belong to the privileged, happy few who have either won the race or have inherited the laurels of the battle. Society does not cease to pay homage to you because you have passed a certain age.

We need, therefore, to recognize the economic basis of our ideology of aging. It is not inevitable for men and women to fear the approach of retirement. The insecurity, loneliness, and loss of self-esteem that we assume to be normative to the aging process are in fact functions of a man-made social structure. In the words of Simone de Beauvoir: "Once we have understood what the state of the aged really is, we cannot satisfy ourselves with higher pensions, decent housing, and organized leisure. It is the whole system that is at issue and our claim cannot be otherwise than radical—change life itself."[21] The negative consequences of aging, de Beauvoir indicates, would be virtually nonexistent. Ultimately death would come, but a person might expect to die without having suffered any degradation.

When a sociologist like Zena Smith Blau observes that there are two instructional structures, the nuclear family and the occupational system, that give "form and meaning to adult existence in modern times," she speaks out of the middle-class bias.[22] De Beauvoir's perspective, which is that of a generalist rather than that of a one-dimensional sociologist, provides a broader vista of possibilities for enhancing the human condition.

New terms often move us to a new consciousness about familiar realities. Our grasp of the process and meaning of aging can be informed by the term "elective years," which was suggested by a newly retired doctor, George A. Perera, writing in *The New York Times* on March 6, 1974. He rejects retirement, although he is giving up his occupational role. It is the continuity of one's life that is important:

> Please let me grow old and call me old, even aged if I need be. I do not want life to be divided into categories with sharp lines between them. I want no disguise or falsification of my advancing years. Life, from its inception until its cessation, is a continuity. I want to be part of it and savor it all, even the inevitability of death.

Old age can be a time when, liberated from the pressures and hang-ups of a youth-oriented society that is driven and harassed by guilt and insecurity, we relish the meaning of life.

Older people should be able to act, live, and take pleasure without having to make every act a moral act. Philip Slater wisely observes that young people are locked into a thought system that they cannot shake off, even though they think of themselves as radical critics of the status quo. Slater writes: "The puritanism of youth displays itself in an inability to act without ideological justification. Every act becomes a moral act."[23] If the young cannot slow down the pace and relax without guilt, the aged, by contrast, ought to be able to savor life quietly and leisurely. They can cultivate the art of living and count the blessings of each day, all the more precious because it is lived more fully. It is the aged who can "live for the day" rather than the young, who rush about transforming the future. De Beauvoir calls our attention to the very moving words Claudel wrote in his *Journal*, at the age of eighty: "Some sigh for yesterday! Some for tomorrow! But you must reach old age before you can understand the meaning, the splendid, absolute, unchallengeable, irreplaceable meaning of the word today!"[24]

Because we still adhere to what Slater calls the "ice-floe approach" to the aged, we are unable to envision the possibilities of secure, meaningful, and even joyous life styles for the aged. We associate status with productivity. We believe everyone must work as long as possible, moonlight if necessary, achieve, and strive. We continue to believe, blindly and tenaciously, that we live in a culture of scarcity and must therefore fight each other for our share of the limited stock of supplies available at any given time. Once again the class variable must be kept in mind. Only the middle and lower classes live in the oppressive ambiance of the scarcity culture. Families that have ascribed status and enjoy financial security live in an economy of abundance. Their destiny is not competition and upward mobility; it is living in the style to which they have been accustomed and maintaining stable and comfortable patterns. They do not struggle to survive or to transcend the standard of living of the parental family. The rich, even if they are idle, are, of course, not without existential anxieties. But they do escape the deprivations of loss of status.

It is not only conceivable but may already be within the grasp of our generation to move from scarcity to abundance. We have sufficient resources and technological capability to provide the good life for all our citizens, regardless of their class or their age grouping. But the belief that the goods of life are in short supply is so strong that we move slowly, if at all, toward a society organized to guarantee total security for all age groups. It is the aged who are the victims, along with members of minority groups, of a society that resists radical social change. We can console ourselves with the knowledge that the means for a good life for all are close at hand. But for the aging of the middle and lower classes, such consolation is too little and too late. If anything, their dissatisfaction and impatience grow all the greater, knowing, as they do, that the means are at hand for an economy of abundance in which they might live with dignity and without loss of self-esteem. For the present, the social ideology of the aging calls for a fairer share of the goods, privileges, and benefits of the social system as now organized. This viewpoint generates pressure on government and competition with other groups. For the aged, time has run out for a program of social reconstruction. The emergency is now; it will do them little or no good to wait. For the country as a whole, however, it is essential to develop a new ideology of the aging and renew our commitment to a society of justice and equality. Ultimate fulfillment for the aging can come only in that day of prophetic peace and right-eousness envisioned by Micah (4:4): "They shall sit every man under his vine and under his fig tree, and none shall make them afraid."

Aging and the "Sabbath" of Man's Life

In concluding this paper, we return to the theme of Judaism and the aging. The prophetic words of Micah remind us of the main thrust in the Jewish tradition toward a belief that the universe is not resistant to the fulfillment of man's hope. There is no reason for any individual or group to compromise their expectation for a life lived to the fullest in a setting of the greatest possible security.

Often religious establishments deny what Marcuse calls "the explosive element" in the teachings they represent.[25] Keeping company with scientists who examine and define the status quo and distance themselves from issues of direction and control, we, in institutional religion, tend, in the words of Marcuse, to "accustom men to a good conscience in the face of suffering and guilt."[26] In reflecting on the religious approach to the situation of the aging in our culture, we might recall the impressive responsibility Marcuse allocates to us: "Where religion still preserves the uncompromised aspirations for peace and happiness, its 'illusions' still have a higher truth value than science which works for their elimination."[27]

In the Jewish view, adumbrated in Scripture and developed more fully in postbiblical Judaism, man is not only encouraged but obliged to hope for salvation. In the vision of the end of days—a time of peace and love—the aged, too, will attain happiness and enjoy the highest esteem, for they represent man in his state of highest self-fulfillment as a child of God.

Life becomes an unending Sabbath for the individual attaining the years of maturity; it persists for him until the day of his death. Nothing captures the essence of the theology of aging in Judaism as does the concept of aging as the Sabbath of the soul with its rich possibilities for self-realization.[28]

It is important to note that work does not have the same meaning in Judaism as in other religious traditions, and therefore ceasing to work and observing the Sabbath has a different rationale and ethic. The distinction between labor during the work week and creative activity on the Sabbath—or in one's so-called retirement years—is vital to the understanding that the Jewish sources contribute to the issue of aging. Work, in the ethos of the Western, middle-class culture, amounts to no less than the primary source of an individual's self-image, his identity, and his self-esteem. A person is valued because he produces; he occupies a status in the economy. Rolelessness or disengagement from the work force is, therefore, dreaded because the individual now suffers from anomie and knows that his community considers him at best an ornament of sentimental interest and, at worse, as a throwaway, used-up object.

In the messianic thought of Judaism (not in the contemporary Jewish community, regrettably), the individual who attains old age is not only not degraded but is honored. The aged can now address themselves to high purposes such as the study of God's word and the purification and refinement of the soul of man. Nothing is lost if man does not have to work; he may still enjoy the Sabbath. As a matter of fact, for him each day is now a Sabbath. The passage in Genesis (3:17) presenting man as toiling life-long to earn his bread has not been taken in Judaism as establishing work as anything like an absolute value. Labor does not serve the function of compensating or atoning for guilt. Necessary as work may be, it is not, as Rabbi Lamm wrote, "an autonomous virtue."[29] It may be true that it is "natural" for man to work—in Genesis 2:15 he is enjoined to till and keep the Garden of Eden—but it is not the necessary condition for salvation.

As the Sabbath is the climax of creation, so the time of maturity represents the highest point of man's development. In the "Sabbath days" of his old age, man has the opportunity not to rest, although he may do that, but to "refresh himself." In the passage in Exodus 31:17 God rests and is refreshed. What God does is paradigmatic for man. Resting, in that passage, signifies cessation from work; being refreshed refers to activity that is creative and active and yields a sense of renewal and inspiration. Ceasing to work does not mean becoming idle or aimless. With leisure comes the opportunity for another kind of activity, the goal of which is the cultivation of one's soul and its potentialities.

What we find in Judaism, therefore, is a magnificent defense of leisure. In the language of the Rabbis, Judaism sanctifies time. You do not "kill" time or "pass" it to fill the void left by retirement. You use it for study, prayer, or contemplation. And if these finer arts do not engage your attention, you fulfill yourself in other ways without feeling inner guilt and without experiencing rejection by the community.

Maimonides wrote a description of the messianic time for those readers inclined toward philosophy and religious study. But his words suggest a perspective and dimension that can be profoundly stimulating to those of us today who seek new values for the aging and who protest the "envy and competition" that presently divide the generations. What, then, are we to do in our leisure and our old age so that we may enjoy self-esteem and possess a sense of salvation? Maimonides wrote:

> The Sages and the prophets did not hope for the coming of the Messiah in order that they might rule over the world, or have dominion over the other nations, or that they might be glorified by other peoples, or in order to eat and drink—but that they be free to engage in the study of Torah and its wisdom, without anyone to oppress them or distract them, so that they might thereby deserve the life of eternity.
>
> In that time (of Messiah) there will be neither famine nor war, neither envy nor competition. Goodness will be available in great abundance, precious things as commonplace as dust. *And the business of the entire world will* be only to know God. . . .[30]

Very few of our aged are endowed with sufficient worldly goods to be able to escape the fate of being stateless, roleless, and virtually homeless. Often they are abandoned by friends and sometimes, by family. They need sensitive pastoral care. They need, too, to sit in a place of dignity with none to make them afraid and with many who will come to them for blessing.

Spiritual Aging

RABBI JACK STERN

I remember coming home after the first day of kindergarten and telling my parents that I had a very pretty teacher—and that she was old. I was 5 then, and I'm sure that my teacher must have been no more than 25. Now that I am 75, when I speak of someone as old, it is usually someone in his or her 90s. When I'm 80, God willing, "old" will be someone in his or her 100s—always that buffer of 20 years.

"Old" is what we are *not yet*. Getting old, yes, but not old. Old is a condition, fixed in one place. Getting older is a process, moving right along. Old is a cesspool, getting older a flowing river.

When we think about the aging process, our first thought is about the onset of limitations, some physical, some cerebral. The next thought then must be how we respond creatively to these limitations. Yet there is another aspect of growing older that is often neglected. This is the spiritual dimension of growing older. The older we get, the more spiritually interesting, and interested, we are capable of becoming. This premise derives from an incident reported by Rabbi Harold Kushner. Apparently one of Agatha Christie's husbands was an archaeologist. A reporter asked the renowned mystery writer, "Miss Christie, what is it like to be married to an archaeologist?" To which she responded, "It's wonderful. The older I get, the more interested he is in me."

The closest we come to the word "spiritual" in the Bible is the famil-

This essay has been adapted from an address delivered at the UAHC Biennial in Orlando, Florida, in December 1999.

iar word *kadosh*—usually translated as "holy, sacred, nonphysical." But in its most original meaning, *kadosh* is understood as "separate, unique, other than the ordinary." God, however differently each of us may conceive of God, is *kadosh*—"Other" with a capital O.

According to our Jewish teachings, each of us is endowed with this capacity to be *kadosh*, which allows us to connect in one way or another with that *kadosh* Other (Leviticus 19:1). In the words of Rabbi Lawrence Kushner, being *kadosh* is "The Self of the I with the Self of the universe," which is what we mean by "spiritual." When we feel weak or diminished or lonely, we can reach out to that *kadosh* Other for strength and support and healing. Or when we are blessed with some good fortune, some gift in life, we can reach out and say, "Thank You, God, that in Your world such good things can happen."

Some psychologists believe that we are naturally endowed with what they call a "spiritual instinct," something inborn. Part of what convinces them is the prevalence of spiritual feelings among young children before they have even been exposed to any religious instruction or indoctrination. In the words of Robert Coles, professor of psychiatry at Harvard Medical School, "These children were revealing an unusual capacity to strive for connection beyond themselves in knowing what their inner world is all about." To use our Jewish vocabulary, they were trying to know what this spiritual *kadosh* connection is all about.

But what happens then? The children grow up into adolescents, and with hormones getting busy and with everything else going on in their lives, spiritual matters are not at the top of their list. They become young adults and then middle-aged, and more and more matters of the inner life give way to matters of the outer one—careers, the needs of their families, making things work, and getting things done. When children have to be given breakfast and sent off to school, there is little time to ponder the essence of life. Scant attention is given to the wonderful mystery of our days and years on this earth when the mystery at hand is how to get the bills paid and still have a balance at the end of the month. And yet one reason for the current wave of spirituality among some of those very same men and women in their middle years is that they have begun to ask what else there is and want to find their way back to that inner *kadosh* world.

But eventually and inevitably come the autumn years, and many of those old responsibilities that once ruled our lives are behind us—somewhat. The children are on their own—somewhat. The clock is no longer such a tyrant—somewhat. There is time left over for other things, including *kadosh* things.

If we are in relatively good health, which most elders today are—even though the machinery of our bodies may be slowing down, even though our memory for names may not be what it once was, even though our physical energy may be springing leaks—our spiritual energy is affected not at all. To the contrary, that spiritual energy may be more ready than ever to be fired up, because now, with time and a slower pace on our side, we are ready for what Zalman Schachter-Shalomi calls "Spiritual Eldering": open to the mysteries we never confronted before, open to questions we never asked before, open to insights we never probed before.

Once, while walking down a street, I noticed a mother and child in front of me. The child had stopped, entranced by a caterpillar inching its way along the side of a leaf. The mother was annoyed and told him to stop dawdling because she had so much to do. In her hurry, she yanked that child away from his *kadosh* moment of spiritual wonderment at God's world.

That's life—we have all been that harried parent. But consider the following, from an essay written by a child in the third grade, entitled "What is a Grandmother?":

> A grandmother is a lady who has no little children of her own. She likes other people's. A grandfather is a man grandmother. Grandmothers don't have to do anything except be there. When they take us for walks, they slow down past things like pretty flowers and caterpillars. They never say 'hurry up.' Grandmothers don't have to be smart, they only have to answer questions like 'Why isn't God married?' and 'How come dogs chase cats?' When they read to us, they don't skip lines or mind if we ask for the same story over again. Everyone should have a grandmother—especially if you don't have a TV, because they are the only grown-ups who have time.

With time on our side, how do we cultivate the art of "Spiritual Eldering"? One answer can be found in an episode from the Torah.

In Genesis 28:10, Jacob is fleeing from his brother Esau. He lies down to sleep with a rock as his pillow, and he has a strange dream. A ladder is standing on the ground, and its top reaches to the heavens. Angels are climbing up and down the ladder. Jacob awakens from his dream and exclaims, "Surely God was in this place, and I did not know it."

This is the itinerary for our own Spiritual Eldering: going up and down that ladder. Up there, when we think the heartwarming thoughts about those who have graced our lives and still do, either in person or in memory. Up there, when we think about all the good times that life smiled on us, and how God's world was good to us. And then back down the ladder, where we come to give something back in return, down here to make good things happen in God's world and in the lives of God's children. Down here is where we give back some of our time, our expertise, and our money. If we need examples, it is reported that the most generous givers to philanthropic causes tend to be from age sixty-five to seventy-four. If we need examples, then it comes from this population of elders who continually provide a major pool of community service *l'takein et haolam*, "to make the world better," whether as volunteers in a hospital, as surrogate grandparents in a classroom, as advisors for start-up business people, or a myriad of other possibilities.

Down here, we are parents to be taken care of—as someone said, it is not role reversal, not the children becoming the parents, but simply the children giving back to the parents who gave so much to them. And again up there, in solitary moments, like spiritual seekers of all ages, we seek a rudder in a storm of illness or financial distress, or the grief of a loss, or the pain of loneliness. And then we come down here again, into our synagogues, for a service of healing or a grief support group to find strength from each other, for a class or Torah study to find strength from the wisdom of a text, or for a Shabbat service to find peace of heart and soul. Being down at the bottom of the *kadosh* ladder is to no longer suffer from the pain of the self-imposed isolation but to reach out to give strength and gain strength. Down here is to make it through a rough day.

And up there, in solitude, we ponder the mysteries and meaning of life and death—including our own life and our own death. Because we who have spent a lifetime affirming life and preserving life, now that the autumn has come, we know that winter is in the offing and that our days on earth will come to an end. So we try to fit together all the pieces of our lifetime, what is sometimes called a "life review": how some of what we did made a difference, and how some of what we failed to do could have made a difference but we didn't know it at the time.

When we were up there putting the pieces together, now and again coming across a broken piece, not yet fixed—a family member or a once good friend, once close and caring, but for whatever reason not so close anymore—these too become part of our life review. When we come back down the ladder, all these broken pieces can help us still fix what deserves to be fixed. We can engage in the serious spiritual business of settling our grudges, seeking forgiveness and granting it, tending to our unfinished business. We needn't wait for Yom Kippur. And so we include in our life review also the values and truths we have come to prize the most, and when we do that, we have, in the words of the Psalmist, "Gotten us a heart of wisdom" (Psalm 90:12).

We carry that wisdom down the ladder with us. In our new spiritual state we can now do what Jews throughout the generations have done. We can compose an ethical will as a message for our children and grandchildren that will outlive our own wintertime. We write about life and love and disappointment and courage and completeness and Jewishness. It may be in the form of a letter, a recording on tape, or simply in words spoken and thoughts expressed on an ordinary day. In whatever form, it will fulfill a major Jewish mandate: "You shall teach them diligently to your children" (Deuteronomy 6:7).

A nurse who had twenty years of experience in a hospice facility reported that the most important lesson she had learned about terminally ill patients is that there is an "easy death" and a "hard death." A hard death is when people struggle emotionally. An easy death is when it happens peacefully, perhaps because their unfinished business has been completed. She said, "All of us have unfinished business. You have it, and I have it, and most patients have it. It is impossible to die in peace unless the unfinished business is put to rest." To which we can add from the wisdom of our tradition that no one needs to wait until the deathbed to finish it (midrash on Psalm 90:12).

And thus the way to our own Spiritual Eldering:

Up there, to utter the silent thank-yous for the blessings of our lives.
Then down here to give something back that will bring blessing into other
lives.
Up there to seek strength and down here to share strength.
Up there to review our lives, and down here to transmit our wisdom and to fix
the broken pieces, and not wait.

And there is yet one more ingredient to that *kadosh* ladder for up there *and* down here. Mary Bray Pipher interviewed a man who had been married sixty-three years and asked him to what he attributed the longevity and stability of his marriage, to which he responded, "It's very simple. Every morning when I get up, I look in the mirror and I say, 'Y'know, you're not such a prize either.'"[1] With all those other ingredients, there is a much needed sense of humor about life and the world and people, and mostly about ourselves. Whoever surrenders that is no longer aging, but just plain old.

Abraham Joshua Heschel wrote about Shabbat, which he calls a palace in time:

> There is a realm of time where the goal is not to have but to
> be, not to own but to share, not to subdue but to be in accord.[2]

Nothing comes as close to a description of spiritual aging. For those in their autumn years, there are all these doors—up there and down here—into this palace of time we call spiritual aging. And once we walk through them, unlike Jacob in the Torah, we shall be able to say, "God is in this place, and I know it very well."

Five Women Spanning
Four Generations

చిం ఎం

Rabbi David Wolfman

The image will stay with me forever. Bubbe Kate, my wife's ninety-five-year-old grandmother, had been living with us for just under a year. When I arrived home from work and entered the kitchen, Jane and Bubbe were standing side by side facing the counter, arms around each other's shoulders. Their backs to me, the glow of the *yahrzeit* candle lit up their silhouettes in gold. "I miss her so much," Bubbe said through her tears. "I do, too," replied Jane. I stood at the door to the kitchen, motionless. I was not going to intrude on this holy moment. My wife and her grandmother were lighting a *yahrzeit* candle for the same woman, the missing generation—Jane for her mother and Bubbe for her daughter. Jane had been lighting the *yahrzeit* candle every year since her mother's death. Bubbe, not very religious, never had before this moment. Yet here they were, in my kitchen, granddaughter teaching grandmother, arm in arm, with loving memories of the same woman. This was beautiful. Clearly it touched the depth of Bubbe's soul. I am convinced, in fact, that the souls of Jane and Bubbe are intertwined.

I am blessed in many ways, by good health, my family, my work, but perhaps the greatest blessing is that I live with five women spanning four generations, ages seven to ninety-five.

The Psalms cry out, "Do not cast me off in old age; when my strength fails, do not forsake me!" (Psalm 71:9). When Bubbe needed a place to live, it took us a nanosecond to agree that she should live with us. Jane and I wanted it to be a family decision. Jennifer, Rachel, and Julie (then twelve, ten, and six) needed to be part of the decision, as it was their house and parents they would be sharing. All of our lives would be impacted. When we told the girls that Bubbe had to move and needed a place to live, it was *their* idea to invite Bubbe to live with us (of course, it was the decision we hoped they would make). For our family, inviting Bubbe to live with us and not "casting her out" was a reflex action: Bubbe needed a place to live, and we had a room to give her. Looking back on that remarkable family discussion, my wife and I are so proud of our daughters for having and knowing how to use that reflex, what I like to call the "mitzvah reflex."

When we made that decision, we also decided that Bubbe would become *part of* our family, not be *apart from* it. That is, Bubbe would not simply be "living" with us. She would be an active member of our family, as it would be her home, too. We were five; we would become six.

And so it is. Bubbe has been a member of our family for over a year, and it has been an even richer experience than we could have possibly imagined. Our tradition teaches that there are three partners in each human being: the father, the mother, and God. When a person honors his or her father and mother, God says, "It is as though I had dwelt among them and they had honored Me" (BT *Kiddushin* 30b). For our family of six, this text rings true every day. When Bubbe moved in, so did yet another presence of the *Shechinah*.[1]

Two times in Torah are we taught about our parents. The first, and most well known, is the Fifth Commandment,

"Honor your father and your mother" (Exodus 20:12;
Deuteronomy 5:16). The second, and somewhat less well
known, is "Let each man be in awe of his parents" (Leviticus
19:3).[2] The Rabbis tell us that revering or holding one's parents in awe is likened to not sitting in your father's chair.
Showing honor to parents includes accepting the responsibility and obligation to care for them, which may include
their health and well-being.[3]

Our daughters did not know this. At their young ages,
they had never studied these texts. Still, somehow deep
inside—with the "mitzvah reflex"—they knew it. We all
knew it. We had been living in our house far longer than
Bubbe has. Still, once Bubbe moved in, it became her home,
too. Our children hold her in awe. She found a chair she likes
in the living room and a seat at the kitchen table. No one else
dares sit there. Not because she would be angry (she would-
n't), but because she likes those seats. They are hers. For our
children, and for my wife and me, it was natural.

People marvel at how I can live happily with five women.
It's easy, actually. It's all in knowing your place in the family.
My home is my palace. Jane is the queen, our daughters are
the princesses, Bubbe is the queen mother (queen grandmother, actually), and I . . . I am their loyal servant!

Are there hardships for us? Certainly. Bubbe is always
cold; consequently, the house is way too hot. Railings had to
be put up around the house and the bathroom had to be
made more accessible. A day care provider (we call her a
"companion") had to be hired. I once had to provide for five;
now with Bubbe and her companion I feed seven. The house
is way too hot. Bubbe needed a subscription to *The New York
Times*, and we recycle too many papers each week. The house
is way too hot. We're finding our public library has a limited

number of large-type romance novels. Did I mention that the house is way too hot?

But these "hardships" come in the form of blessings. I hope I am around when I'm ninety-five—and in good health, just like Bubbe. I pray to God that there will be people (specifically my great-grandchildren) who love me enough to live in constant subtropical temperatures. I hope I can learn from my grandchildren just as Bubbe learns from Jane . . . and I pray to God that my great-grandchildren will still be able to love, smile, laugh with, hug, kiss, and learn from me.

"*Ashreinu mah tov chelkeinu*—how beautiful is our portion!" (BT *Yoma* 87b). It is my fortune, my honor, to live with these five wonderful women. I am a constant witness to the transmission of values, stories, and a weaving relationship, all of which fill our home with holiness, love, and learning.

Bubbe says that moving into our house was like moving into her own. What a compliment. Bubbe goes to all of our children's concerts, plays, and science fairs. She can't see them or hear them. But our kids can see and hear her. She told me that she goes just for that reason: so they know that she is there.

Still, at ninety-five, Bubbe wakes up each morning and has breakfast with the family, walks up and down the block twice a day, or during inclement weather, takes thirty minutes to walk the interior perimeter of our house, only to begin her calisthenics. I try to miss this part, as it depresses (read: inspires) me. She touches the floor with her palms twenty-five times and then stretches. (I can't even touch my toes!) After she exercises her body, she exercises her mind. She writes. (She's legally blind . . . but Jane and I think she is selectively blind. She can spot chocolate a mile away!) She writes the numbers one through ten in numerical form and spells them out, and then proceeds to write down every person's name in her family (daughter, grandchildren, great-grandchildren, all their spouses) along with their *birthdays!* She spends her afternoons reading her romance novels from the library, doing the *Boston Globe's* crossword puzzle with her companion, and playing Scrabble, her passion. The Scrabble set (Jane bought her special larger bright white tiles) is always near the table. Our next-door neighbor, Grace (a young woman in her seventies), comes over each day at two o'clock to play three games of Scrabble. Jane and I take delight not only in their friendship, but in the fact that our daughters see that Bubbe has a life outside of the five of us.

Bubbe holds a bachelor of science degree in government and law from NYU. She played for the NYU women's varsity basketball team—we have the newspaper clippings to prove it! Recently, when preparing her taxes and other assorted paperwork, I came across her NYU diploma rolled up in a rubber band—she has a great collection of rubber bands.

"Bubbe," I said, "let me frame this."

"This? Why? I don't need it."

"Bubbe, please allow me. I want the girls to see what their great-grandmother has accomplished."

"Whatever." It was all the approval I needed.

Bubbe is a fifty-year breast cancer survivor and has just completed six weeks of radiation for another bout of breast cancer. The diagnosis came just after her ninety-fifth birthday. The decision to treat came easily to her: She is, after all, healthy. "This is going to be hard," we thought. "This is going to be especially hard on the kids," we thought. How wrong we were.

For six weeks, Jane or I drove her to the hospital for her daily radiotherapy treatment. Jane and I are also abundantly blessed with the fact that Jane's brother and sister-in-law live just around the corner and that we have the best friends on earth. When Jane or I could not drive to the hospital, they were there . . . not to drive Jane's grandmother, but to go with their friend, Bubbe.

As soon as she got home, it was back to her morning routine. She didn't skip a beat.

Hard for our children? On the contrary. She has taught us all valuable lessons through her cancer and her healing. You go into something strong, you come out strong. Exercise your body and then immediately exercise your mind. Don't let anything stop you.

Our daughters see that aging is a part of living. Our daughters know that while you may lose some facilities as you age, *inside every old person is every person they have ever been.*[4] Inside Bubbe, inside this ninety-five-year-old great-grandmother, is a child, daughter, sister, adolescent, girlfriend, basketball player, student of law and government, wife, mother, and so much more. All of those experiences are inside of her.

One Shabbat afternoon, our eldest daughter came home from a bar mitzvah reception, her face stained with tears. She sat on my lap and silently cried on my shoulder. It seemed that a boy had said something that hurt her. My first instinct was to find that boy and . . . but then I realized that my thirteen-year-old teenager was, after all, sitting on my lap, and although crying, hugging me. Not bad!

Bubbe was sitting next to us on the sofa. "What's the matter?" she asked.

I asked Jen if I could tell her. She nodded.

"A boy said a hurtful thing to Jen, and she's sad."

"Humph!" said Bubbe, with an upward motion of her hand. Jen and I were startled by this. And then I understood.

"Bubbe," I asked, what were boys like when you were in middle school eighty-two years ago?"

"Boys? Much the same as they are now and will always be: JERKS!"

Jennifer's eyes opened wide, and a smile grew across her face from ear to ear. She gave me a hug, gave Bubbe a hug, and went off.

A week later while I was traveling, I called home to say goodnight. When Jen took the phone, I asked her about her day. It was "cool." She went over to this boy's house and played with his new puppy.

"But Jen, isn't this the guy who said those things last weekend?"

"Yeah, Dad," she said, "but you heard Bubbe. All boys are jerks. Now I know that, and we can be friends." Bubbe, not I, had healed her.

Rachel, our eleven-year-old, recently had to prepare and deliver a speech on a "Special Person." She chose Bubbe. Rachel asked Bubbe if she would come to school so that she could introduce her to the class. Bubbe's visit to the fifth grade allowed the entire class to meet and speak with this amazing woman. Rachel's teacher still mentions Bubbe to the class.

At the end of the speech, Rachel gave Bubbe a copy of her "Special Person" speech, typed in a very large font size. Are there benefits for bringing in those you love to live with you? Our daughter, on her own, knew that her great-grandmother would enjoy having a copy of her "Special Person" speech, and she also knew that she couldn't read it unless it was enlarged. Our pride in her is overwhelming.

Our youngest, Julie, was doing a project on ancestors. She had to find out where her family came from. In her class, there are several first- and second-generation Americans. Julie is fourth generation. For her report she brought in the first generation—Bubbe! How proud she was to show off her great-grandma! How proud Bubbe was to be shown off!

And Bubbe? She still glows when she repeats the story of her outings to elementary school as "Show-and-Tell." I still don't know who gained more—great-granddaughters or great-grandmother.

Having Bubbe live with us is great for Jane. Through her daily relationship with Bubbe, I am sure she feels more connected with her mother (z"l).[5] In many ways, the relationship between Jane and Bubbe—granddaughter and grandmother—helps to keep her memory alive. Jane very rarely wears the ring I gave her upon our engagement. Not because she doesn't like it—she loves it. Instead, she now wears the ring her mother left her. It was her mother's engagement ring, and before that it was Bubbe's. I really don't mind that the engagement ring I gave to Jane sits in the safe. It's not going anywhere (except to one of our daughters one day, please God). She still loves the ring (and me). I know that in wearing her mother's ring, which was her mother's mother's ring, she is able to keep her mother's memory alive and, *at the same time,* she knows Bubbe sees her wearing it, and that gives both of them joy. So much energy flows through that stone.

Jane is the nurturing caregiver and fun-loving grandchild at the same time. She can flip back and forth between tending to Bubbe's health needs and hygiene—with an abundance of modesty and respect—and being the fun-loving granddaughter who wants only to play with her Grandma. One of the "pictures" I carry in my mind is the time Jane and Bubbe were standing forehead to forehead, pointer finger touching the other's pointer finger, grinning from ear to ear while talking in the secret family "R" language Grandpa Ben (z"l) made up when they were all kids.

Having Bubbe live with us is good for me. I had an adult relationship with only one of my grandmothers. I miss her very much. I actually don't call Bubbe "Bubbe." I call her "Grandma." My children have noticed and have asked me why. I tell them it's because Bubbe is like my Grandma; she fills that void in my life. I love my relationship with Bubbe. I especially love being able to honor my wife's mother's mother. I loved driving her to the hospital (though I wished she didn't have to go) and spending the time alone with her. I enjoy keeping up with the stock market (she's actually teaching me a lot!) so that I can come home and tell her, "Grandma, the market went up 120 points," something I know she already knows but enjoys hearing it just the same. I love holding her hand as we walk. I love when she places her arm in mine. I am proud of her.

Having Bubbe live with us is also good for Bubbe. She is ninety-five years old and is a vital part of our family. She has taken some household chores upon herself. She is the recycling maven, each morning taking yesterday's *Boston Globe* and *New York Times* downstairs to the recycling bins. She also dries dishes. I enjoy washing the dishes while she dries. It's a time to talk. Working together, each contributing to our household. It has a calming effect. She is not just biding her time and letting life pass her by. Not Bubbe.

When I was a child, there was an old man who lived down the block from me. I would watch him walk so very slowly up and down the street while I was playing or riding my bicycle. I never said anything to him. I was afraid of him. He was the oldest man I had ever seen.

I love that our children's friends run in and out of our

house, see Bubbe sitting in her chair, shout, "Hi, Bubbe!" and give a friendly smile and wave. Some even come over and kiss her hello and good-bye. I love that our children's friends know that Bubbe is a part of our family and that they feel comfortable around her. I love when our friends invite us to dinner and assume—even look forward to—the fact that Bubbe will be coming, too. I love standing in our Shabbat Circle, holding hands, and seeing that our children's friends are not afraid to hold her hand.

Friday nights are special. Most Friday nights we have another family over for dinner. Very often it is Jane's brother, sister-in-law, and their children (two more of Bubbe's great-grandchildren—she has thirteen in all). We begin our Shabbat ritual by standing in a circle, arm in arm, singing Shabbat songs until we are all ready to continue. We then bless the children and exchange our family kisses.

When we gather around the Shabbat table, each person takes a turn placing a coin in the *tzedakah* box and has the opportunity to share something of which they are proud or for which they are grateful. Each week, for over a year, and without fail, Bubbe says the same thing:

"I just want to say how happy I am to be here with all of you."

She means it. That's why, I believe, she says it each week, as if we have never heard it before. She truly is thankful that she is able to be with us. I don't think she means just *physically* being with us; I think she means *being* with us: she is present *and* a presence. We cannot imagine our family without her.

⚬ⱳⱳⱳ⚬

Beyond Guilt:
What We Owe Our Aging Parents—
A Perspective from Tradition

RABBI DAYLE A. FRIEDMAN

Rabbi Shimon ben Yochai said: ". . . The most difficult of
all mitzvot is 'Honor your father and your mother. . . .'"
Tanchuma, Eikev, 2

We are pacing in the family waiting room. Each of us has our eyes on
the door to the intensive care unit and an ear affixed to a cell phone. My
siblings and I are each trying to be in two places at once. We are in the
hospital attending to my stepfather, who has just had a serious heart
attack. And we are trying, by long-distance telephone, to manage our
individual lives, thousands of miles away. We are talking to toddlers,
cheering overwhelmed spouses, canceling appointments, juggling work
commitments, and feeling generally awful as we wrestle with our decisions about leaving. My brother decides to go home after two days so that
he can be with his son on the first day of kindergarten. I choose to forego
accompanying my two-year-old twins to their first day of day care. My
stepbrother decides to miss yet another day of income from his private
practice so that he can be with the folks for Shabbat. We know that whenever we leave it will be too soon for my parents and my sister, our only
local sibling; they are grateful for every moment of presence, encourage-
ment, and advocacy. And however long we stay is too long for our children, who are too young to understand, and for our partners, who are
heroically doing the work of two parents.[1]

According to a Yiddish saying, "With one *tuchis* you can't dance at two
weddings." With our finite time, energy, and finances, we nonetheless try

to find a way, if not to be in two places at once, at least to come close. When we can't do it, we feel guilty and disappointed in ourselves. My siblings and I are confronting the painful dilemmas of multiple and often competing obligations, and the choices we are forced to make are often wrenching. Like so many others in our life situation, we desperately need wisdom. We want to know what we owe our aging parents and how we are to navigate the treacherous terrain of finitude—ours and theirs—and seemingly irreconcilable competing demands.

When we think about seeking counsel from our tradition, we imagine that we will find only absolute commandments about filial piety, such as "Honor your father and your mother" in the Ten Commandments. We are afraid that Jewish law and values will merely validate our already overpowering sense of guilt for not doing, or being, enough for our parents. Actually, our Jewish tradition is far more nuanced, realistic, and sagacious. Judaism offers a perspective on relationships between adult children and their parents that can provide us with compassionate, pragmatic moral guidance. Our tradition urges respectful, attentive care, on the one hand, and on the other, recognizes and supports accepting the limits of what adult children can do. This essay will examine texts that outline our basic obligations to our aging parents and will also analyze the limits on our obligations and the relevance of these texts for our contemporary quandaries as we try to move beyond guilt.

The Dimensions of the Caregiving Demand

Though the details of my family's situation are unique, experiencing increasing demands to care for elderly parents is not. This is due in part to demographic and sociological realities, as well as emotional and financial issues. The blessings of medical advances and increased longevity have created the challenge of prolonged periods of dependency among older people. Elders may be able to live for decades despite considerable frailty and dependency. The decrease in the birthrate and rise in mobility in the Jewish community mean that there are fewer caregivers available to do the formidable task of caring for aging parents. Many people assume that children of elderly parents today are less dutiful than those in previous generations. On the contrary, far from abandoning their parents, most adult children earnestly want to care for them and are committed to doing whatever they can. However, as in my family, the obligations to aging parents are not the only demands upon most caregivers. They are simultaneously pulled in many directions by the competing and compelling claims of child rearing, spouses, and career.[2]

Like me and my siblings, most caregivers feel guilty some or even all of the time. Not only are caregivers' resources stretched over multiple demands, but the nature of the caregiving task itself easily induces guilt, as an old Yiddish folktale teaches:

> A mother bird was carrying her three babies across a river. As she carried the first baby in her beak high above the river, she asked her child, "When I am old, will you do the same for me?" "Of course, Mother," replied the baby. "It will be my honor." The mother bird dropped the baby into the river saying simply, "You're a liar!"
>
> As she carried the second baby, the mother again asked, "When I am old, will you do the same for me?" The second baby bird replied as the first, and the mother bird dropped it, too, into the river.
>
> When she carried the third baby across the river, the mother bird asked it, "When I am old, will you carry me across the river as I am carrying you now?" The baby bird answered dolefully, "Oh no, Mother, when you are old, I will have children of my own, and I shall have to carry them across the river. I won't be able to carry you, as well." The mother bird replied, "You are my darling child, for you have told the truth." She carried this baby to the other side of the river and gently put him down.[3]

As the tale illustrates, we can never repay our parents for the care they gave to us. Moreover, the nature of care for a child is different than care for a parent. While a child naturally grows toward greater competency and less dependency, our parents are likely to need *more* care over time. Caregiving for aging parents has no end point besides death. It is difficult to feel we are successful at caring for dependent parents, since they usually do not "get better."

Caregiving for parents is emotionally complex, since it challenges the order of the relationship that we've known up to that point. We are used to our parents being "in charge" and to their taking care of us. Turning the tables in these regards can be provocative at best. In relationships where there has been conflict, strain, or estrangement, the new situation might create an opening for healing, but it can also dredge up old wounds. Painful past experiences may limit the ways in which an adult child is able or willing to care for a parent.

Caregivers struggle to "do the right thing," to successfully traverse unfamiliar territory without a map. We look to our tradition to replace guilt, which can be paralyzing, with orienting values, which can fortify and direct us.

Fundamental Obligations of Adult Children toward Aging Parents

The Torah includes two basic commandments regarding children's obligations toward their parents. The first of these is the Fifth Commandment: "Honor your father and your mother that your days may be long upon the land that *Adonai* your God is giving you" (Exodus 20:12). In the Holiness Code, the obligation is stated differently: "You shall each revere your mother and your father, and keep My sabbaths: I, *Adonai*, am your God" (Leviticus 19:3).[4]

It is interesting to note that in both instances, the obligations toward parents are linked directly to our relationship to God. This feature can be interpreted in various ways. Clearly, the connection to God underscores the importance of the mitzvah. Perhaps the texts draw an analogy between our obligations to parents and our obligations toward God. One further characteristic of these texts is worth noting. The Fifth Commandment is the only one among the Ten Commandments that promises a reward for obeying it. The presence of the promised reward might hint at the difficulty of observing this mitzvah. That the promised reward is long life suggests that caring for parents fits into a system of intertwined relationships. We care for our parents in the hope that we will be blessed to live to a ripe old age and that we will be cared for by our children when we reach that point.

Although we are commanded by the Torah to love God and to love our neighbors, interestingly, neither of these commandments requires that we *love* our parents. In fact, the Torah is silent about how we must feel about them. Perhaps acknowledging the complexity of parent-child relationships, the Torah commands us only to respectfully lend assistance to our parents.

Rabbinic interpretation assumes that even seemingly redundant passages are in the text to teach us something important. Thus, the Rabbis suggest that these similar mitzvot teach us about two discrete and fundamental aspects of our obligations to our parents.

> Our Rabbis taught: What is reverence [*mora*] and what is honor [*kavod*]? Reverence means that he [the son] must neither stand nor sit in his [father's] place, nor contradict his words, nor tip the scale against him. Honor means that he must give him food and drink, clothe and cover him, and lead him in and out.
>
> BT *Kiddushin* 31b

Reverence, *mora*, is preserving our parents' dignity. This commandment relates to the attitude of respect that is due our parents. The text identifies and prohibits behaviors that might compromise the parent's dignity. Even if our roles have shifted and we are now caring for our parents, we are called to allow them to keep their place. We must not usurp their position of respect or authority. We must not take advantage of them. And we must not make decisions that fail to respect their wishes.

A daughter is acting with *mora* when she makes a medical decision for her mother who is no longer able to do so and decides based on her mother's values, goals, and previously stated preferences. The son whose very frail father desperately wants to remain at home can also demonstrate *mora*. Here, *mora* may mean respecting his father's wishes, even if the son is worried that his father will be lonely, and helping his father to hire help so that he can safely remain home. An adult child can show *mora* to a parent in a nursing home by making sure to include him or her in *simchah*s (joyous occasions), such as a grandchild's bar mitzvah, and even *tzures* (sad occasions), such as a funeral for a family member. Rejoicing and crying with their families help frail elders to know they are still part of life. These and other similar acts of respect grant reverence to parents who have lost much; they allow them to maintain their place.

In contrast to *mora*, which is attitudinal, honor, *kavod*, revolves around providing for our parents' material and concrete needs. This mitzvah obligates us to ensure that our parents have adequate shelter, food, clothing, and transportation. It is our responsibility to see that they are well cared for. There is a debate in the sources about the issue of financial responsibility. Some authorities hold that a child must pay for a parent's needs, while others argue that the child is obliged to make sure the needs are met but can use the parent's money to pay for this.[5]

Nearly every adult child caring for an aging parent has had the opportunity to provide him or her with *kavod*, in the sense of providing for concrete needs. Every time a daughter takes her mother to a medical appointment or shopping, she is offering *kavod*. Each act of advocating for the needs of a father who is in a nursing home is an opportunity to provide *kavod*. Every invitation for an aging parent to come to Shabbat dinner can also be an act of *kavod*, as can helping him or her write checks for monthly bills. Of course, long-distance caregiving makes providing *kavod* particularly challenging. Regular visits, taking responsibility for particular aspects of a parent's care, and helping to coordinate others who provide care can all be part of offering *kavod* to parents who live far away.

The Rabbis emphasize that the *manner* in which we carry out our obligations is as important as the *fact* of doing so.

> Abimi the son of Rabbi Abahu taught: A son may feed his father pheasant, and [yet] be driven from the world [to come]; he may chain him to the millstone, and merit the world-to-come thereby.
>
> BT *Kiddushin* 31a–b

Rashi explains that grudgingly providing material abundance is not enough. Though he might appear to be giving his parent treatment fit for a king, the person who feeds his father pheasant is punished because "he displays a mean spirit as he feeds him." On the other hand, being unable to wrest a parent from scarcity is not a sin. The son who chains his father to the millstone makes his father work in order to help sustain the family. According to Rashi, he is rewarded because "he honors him by speaking good and comforting words, imposing the labor gently by showing him . . . that they could not sustain themselves without his labor." Difficult though it may be, we are called to care for our parents with an attitude of deference, willingness, and compassion.

One additional mitzvah from the Torah guides our relationships with aging parents. This commandment concerns our relationships with all older people, not just our own parents: "You shall rise before the gray-haired person and grant glory [v'hadarta p'nei zakein] to the face of the elderly" (Leviticus 19:32). Danny Siegel translates the phrase v'hadarta p'nei zakein, "allow the beauty, glory, and majesty of their faces to emerge."[6] According to this reading, our obligation toward our elders is not just to treat them with respect, but to enable them to experience joy, meaning, and pride. This commandment is in some ways even more demanding than the others, for it requires assisting elders to have what Bill Thomas, who has pioneered revolutionary changes in nursing home care, calls "a life worth living."[7] On the other hand, it is comforting that this commandment is really societal, for the obligation of hidur p'nei zakein is upon all Jews toward all elders. This text thus suggests that the burden of caring for elders belongs to the whole community, not just to adult children.

Competing Claims:
Limits on Our Obligations to Aging Parents

Our tradition understands that adult children may confront the obligation to care for their parents at the same time that they are caring for partners and children, as well as working to support their families. Our Rabbis are also realistic about the limits imposed on a child's caregiving capacity by the parent's condition, as well as by problematic relationships. The obligation to aging parents is qualified by these factors.

Marriage and Children

As important as are our obligations to our parents, they are superceded by the preciousness of the marital bond. Honoring our parents and caring for them must not, according to the Rabbis, endanger marital harmony. So, for example, Maimonides teaches that one spouse must not impose his or her parents on the other if being with them is conflictual or unpleasant.

> If a man says to his wife, "I don't want your father and mother and brothers and sisters to come to my home," his wishes are heeded, but she shall go to them when it becomes a hardship for them. She shall go to her father's home once a month and on every Festival. And they shall not visit her, except if this is a hardship for her, e.g., she is ill or in labor, for a person is not forced to have others enter his dominion. And, if she were to say, "I don't want your mother and sisters (to come to me) and I shall not live in the same courtyard with them, for they are bad to me and cause me grief," her wishes are to be heeded, for a person is not compelled to have others dwell in his or her domain.[8]

Note that one is still obligated to remain in contact with and care for one's parents, but to do so in a way that will not compromise *sh'lom bayit*, domestic peace.

When we are torn between attending to the needs of parents and those of partners and children, this approach suggests we give priority to our partners and children. For example, when Lee's ninety-six-year-old father, Sol, fell in the nursing home and needed to go to the hospital to have a cut on his head stitched, she was not able to go with him. Her husband, Morrie, was hospitalized for a heart attack on the very same day, and her first obligation was to be with him. Of course, placing priority on one set of obligations does not release us from the other. So, in this case, Lee visited Sol two days later when Morrie had stabilized, but in the meantime made sure that her nephew went to visit him that very day.[9]

The needs faced by caregivers often seem limitless, but adult children are mortal, finite beings. Our tradition recognizes these limits. We are encouraged to work to strike a balance. Although our sources are filled with stories exalting exemplary, self-sacrificing care for parents,[10] there is also a sense that we can only do the best we can.

The Adult Child's Well-Being

Caring for a parent is demanding and can be exhausting, as well. But, according to our tradition, it should not be allowed to be destructive to a person's mental or physical health. Maimonides, for example, specifically suggests that there may come a time when an adult child is no longer able to directly provide the care a parent needs.

> If one's father or mother should become mentally disordered, he should try to treat them as their mental state demands, until they are pitied by God [they die]. But if he finds he cannot endure the situation because of their extreme madness, let him leave and go away, deputing others to care for them properly.[11]

It seems likely that Maimonides is referring to parents who are suffering from dementia. In this situation, he teaches, adult children may reach a point where they can no longer stand to be the hands-on caregivers of their parents. Significantly, the criterion for when that point is reached is the adult children's *subjective* experience. Only the adult children can say when they have reached their limit.

As before, the child's responsibility for the parent remains. What has changed is that he or she is empowered to arrange for others to provide that care. Although he does not clearly state it, it would seem that Maimonides would expect the child to continue to provide *mora*, respect for the parent's dignity, even while the obligation for *kavod* is being carried out indirectly.

Maimonides' teaching is particularly relevant to those caring for parents suffering from dementia, such as Alzheimer's disease. In the early stages of the disease, caregivers may be able to support parents with regular phone calls and reminders about daily tasks, such as taking medicines. As dementia progressively robs individuals of their faculties, their children may find themselves stressed beyond their limits. Both the need for constant supervision and the very intimate care that those in the later stages of dementia require are often unbearable for family caregivers.[12] Maimonides teaches us that we are allowed to respect the limits of our endurance engendered by our parents' condition. Placing a demented parent in the care of others, in his or her own home, in an assisted living facility, or in a nursing home, is an agonizing choice, but one that Maimonides would seem to endorse for those who no longer have the emotional or physical resources to provide the care themselves.

We also learn from the Rabbis that we may need to withdraw from direct care in the case of abusive or highly conflicted relationships.

> It is best that a father and a son separate if they quarrel with each other, for much pain is caused; and I do not mean only the pain of the father or teacher, but even the pain of the son.[13]

In this instance, the medieval moral text, *Sefer Chasidim*, teaches that caring for a parent should be done at a distance if coming into contact produces arguments that are painful and destructive for the adult child. We can assume that the text is not addressing the kind of periodic disagreements or conflicts that are part of the fabric of normal relationships, but rather conflicts and behavior that are truly pathological. We are obligated to preserve our own wholeness, as Hillel so aptly taught, "If I am not for myself, who will be for me?" (*Pirkei Avot* 1:14).

Although we tend to think of caregiving in terms of the child's obligations toward the parents, our tradition teaches that the parent has obligations, as well. The parent is forbidden to make things harder upon the child or to be overly demanding.

> Although we are commanded (regarding honoring parents), a person is forbidden to add to the burden upon his child, and to be particular regarding his honor, lest he bring them to a stumbling block, rather, he should be forgiving, and ignore [behavior that is not strictly in keeping with the mitzvah], for when a parent is forgiving regarding his or her honor, his or her honor is preserved (a parent has the right to forego the honor due him). One who strikes an adult child is to be ostracized, for he has transgressed the commandment "Do not place a stumbling block before the blind."[14]

Maimonides wisely counsels the parent who is the recipient of care to be forbearing. He realizes that approaching one's children with an attitude of generosity and forgiveness is more likely to yield the desired result of respectful treatment than critically judging their every action. A parent must not look for what a child has failed to do; the parent who acknowledges and appreciates the child's care will be the richer for it.

Our tradition recognizes that one's obligations to provide care are brought into question in cases where there has been abuse or mistreatment by the parent. While some sources suggest that the child's obligation is in force even if a parent has wronged him or her, others suggest that one is obligated only where the parent has repented, where there has been acknowledgment of the wrong and restitution. The teaching of Joseph Caro, the author of the *Shulchan Aruch*, the Code of Jewish Law, seems to be contradicted by that of Moses Isserles, the author of the gloss on that text.

> CODE: A bastard is obliged to honor and fear his father; even if his father is an evil-doer and a violator of the law, he must honor him and stand in awe of him.
> GLOSS: And some say that one is not obliged to honor one's wicked father unless he repents.[15]

While Caro states that a parent's sinful behavior does not limit a child's obligations, Isserles suggests that a child is not obligated toward a parent who has transgressed laws or limits and failed to take responsibility for his or her actions. One way of harmonizing these views is to suggest that a child of an abusive parent is called to at least avoid doing anything active to hurt or dishonor a parent, but may not be obligated to provide direct care or take active measures to honor that parent. Thus, a child who has survived sexual abuse by her father could feel she has done the right thing by avoiding contact with him, while a son whose father is in recovery from alcoholism and has asked for his forgiveness might feel called to attend to his care needs.

Conclusion

Adult children of aging parents face a daunting task. Not only are the needs of aging parents extensive, but our responsibilities toward them are also enormous. Jewish tradition helps us to find our way through the painful tensions between our obligations to our aging parents and our responsibilities to our spouses, our children, and ourselves. The texts and values we have explored affirm both our powerful obligations and our very real limits and humanity. Our caregiving can be guided by the teaching of Rabbi Tarfon: "It is not your obligation to complete the task, but neither are you free to desist from it" (*Pirkei Avot* 2:21). Our tradition thus urges us to stretch mightily in bringing our physical presence and our spiritual and material resources to the work of caring for our aging parents, but to forgive ourselves for not being able to do it perfectly. This, ultimately, can help us to move beyond guilt and into empowered responsibility.

Honor Thy Mother and Thy Father

———————————

ᏟᏋ ᏰᎧ

Janice London Bergman

As I sit beside my Dad in curtained cubicle 12 of the emergency room, I watch in fascination as my Dad's chest heaves up and down with what looks like great effort. His heart monitor is erratic, his blood tests show yet another bout with sepsis (a serious bacterial infection in his blood), his renal system isn't functioning well, and he may have pneumonia. Considering he experienced the same symptoms exactly seven weeks ago in a different hospital ER, this appears very serious to me.

This latest ambulance race to the ER has given me cause to pause and reflect over the last twelve years. I think about the mantra that I have been using throughout this time, "Honor thy mother and thy father." I sit beside him and analyze whether in all the instances, when I have been "put to the test" as the caregiver, I have honored them and still been true to myself. I know it is a risky exercise, but I still do it. My analysis, fortunately, turns out to be positive. Others in my situation, unfortunately, are not as lucky.

It is easy to sit in judgment of what a caregiver decides to do on behalf of his or her mom or dad; but not until you, as that adult child, have walked in the same shoes, can you begin to recognize the difficulty of the situation. It is hard putting yourself in your parent's place in order to "think" the way they would as a means of guiding your decision making. It is even tougher when the decision you have made on their behalf turns out to be a bad one. Worse, yet, when you must accept a decision that a third party has made, without your input, and it turns out horrific. But those scenarios are all part of what one lives with as a parental caregiver.

It was January 1994 when, by virtue of a long-distance phone call from Florida at 3:00 A.M., I was thrust into the role of my parents' caregiver—a role I neither wanted, was prepared for, nor had the training for. But then, most of us in the "sandwich generation" have similar stories and never asked for the added responsibility.

Their story begins when they moved from Chicago to Florida upon retirement. Dad was using a wheelchair, Mom a walker. They had a life filled with friends, card games, dinner parties, and theater. And, in spite of her limitations, Mom was Dad's full-time caregiver: her raison d'être. Then the unthinkable happened . . . she fell. That was the beginning of the end of their independence, freedom, and life as they had known it. When the caregiver no longer can care for her- or himself, the house of cards collapses. A new phase began for them and for me.

Mother went into a nursing home rehabilitation center; Dad stayed in their condo. I tried to manage their lives long-distance. Round-the-clock care was obtained for him, which sometimes worked and sometimes didn't. After five months of this arrangement, we gave in to the impossible odds. Dad joined mom in the nursing home.

I continued handling their finances, the difference being that I now wrote two additional checks each month for the cost of their nursing home. This additional amount was $7200. Before too long, I had the sad task of exercising my "power of attorney" and selling their condo, dissolving all of their household goods and locking the doors on the first home they had ever owned. Next came the sale of their car; followed by the cashing in of their IRAs, their stocks, and their savings and checking accounts. All this to pay the monthly costs of the nursing home.

Within two years their assets were completely "spent down," and I applied for Florida Medicaid Long-Term Care Benefits on their behalf. After providing the Medicaid Long-Term Care office with reams and reams of paperwork and documentation, they rendered their opinion: Dad was accepted, and they agreed to pay for the cost of his nursing home care; Mom was not. They stated that because she did not truly need the care of a skilled nursing home, she was not eligible for the benefits. So, for the first time in fifty-four years of marriage, my parents were forced to live in separate places. She went into an assisted living facility; he stayed at the nursing home. What happened to my parents was cruel and inhumane. It didn't seem fair or just that some bureaucratic rule could so easily rob them of growing old together.

And so we marked another phase in my parents' lives, which continued for several years.

I moved my parents to the Washington, D.C. area in 1998. That decision did not come quickly or easily. I tried to look at every aspect of their lives and realized that I could better monitor their health if they lived nearby. "Honor thy mother and thy father" played over and over in my mind during the difficult task of their physical move, but we accomplished it without too many crises.

They still lived in separate places, but I was available to

drive her to visit him. Their lives became more meaningful because of my husband's and my continual involvement in their lives. My parents again were having wonderful memories: their grandchildren and four great-grandchildren visiting them on a regular basis; Pesach at my house, for the first time in more than a decade; other holiday celebrations; birthday parties; barbecues—all the pleasures of family life.

The pièce de résistance occurred in early 2000, when Allan and I celebrated our tenth anniversary. We renewed our marriage vows in our synagogue followed by dinner and dancing. We honored my parents in front of our family and friends as we announced their approaching sixtieth wedding anniversary. And seeing them on the dance floor in their wheelchairs dancing along with everyone else was worth a million dollars. They smiled, they glowed, and they enjoyed the celebration as much as we did.

Six short weeks later, my mother died, never having had the opportunity to celebrate that special anniversary. I felt comforted, however, in the knowledge that her life had been extended by the move here. And, I certainly knew it had been more meaningful. I believed, as we lay her to rest, that I had truly "honored her."

Yet another phase was entered. Did we buy my parents another week, a month, a year, four years? I don't really know, but I do know they were able to have a better "quality of life." Their lives have been prolonged, and it has been meaningful. A wonderful accomplishment!

I further know that, whether Dad makes it this time or not, I have honored them throughout the entire process. And, for that I feel blessed.

⟨∞∞⟩

Who Pays? The Talmudic Approach
to Filial Responsibility

RABBI MICHAEL CHERNICK

The Text: BT *Kiddushin* 31b–32a

Text: Our Rabbis taught: What constitutes respect for parents
and what constitutes honoring them?

Commentary: In Exodus 20:12 it states: "Honor your father and your
mother that you may lengthen your days on the land that the Eternal,
your God, has given you." In Leviticus 19:3 we find, "Each person shall
respect [lit., fear] his/her mother and father, and you shall keep My sabbaths." These verses are the background for the question above.

Text: Respect is observed by not standing in the parent's usual
place, nor sitting where they normally sit, by not contradicting the parent's words, and by not interfering in a parent's dispute with others.

Commentary: Noninterference in a dispute between a parent and others is interpreted differently by various commentators. Rashi, the
Talmud's most famous interpreter, held that a child should not side
against the parent. The *Shulchan Aruch*, the major code of Jewish law,

This lecture was originally given as part of the Sunday at the College Series, February 23, 1986
in New York.
Reprinted, with changes, from *The Journal of Aging and Judaism* 1, no. 2 (spring/summer
1987): 109–17.

suggests that a child should not even support the parent's position in an argument with others. This latter view was prompted by the sense that taking the opponent's side was not different from contradicting the parent. Hence, noninterference had to mean something other than siding against one's parent in a dispute. The view is very interesting, and we shall return to it in our analysis of this text as a whole.

Text: Honoring one's parents is observed by helping them to eat and drink, clothing and covering them, and helping them to go in and out.

A question was raised by the Rabbis: Who pays for this? [lit., From whom?]. R. Judah said, "The child." R. Nathan b. Oshaiah said, "The parent."

Commentary: The question relates to the commandment of honor since, as it was defined, it entails expenditures for food and clothing. Obviously, the parent who needs to be fed, clothed, and accompanied by another is of fairly advanced age. The "child" is an adult child, since minors are not obliged to observe the commandments according to Jewish law.

Text: The Rabbis ruled according to the opinion that the parent must pay [in answer to a legal query raised by] R. Jeremiah. There are those that say [in answer] to R. Jeremiah's son.

This ruling was challenged by the following source: The Torah states, "Honor your father and mother," and Proverbs states, "Honor the Eternal with your wealth" (Proverbs 3:9). Just as "honor" in regard to God means through monetary expenditure, so "honor" in regard to a parent means through monetary expenditure.

If the parent is to pay, in what way does the child observe the requirement to pay for his/her parent's honor? [The answer is:] through time given up from gainful pursuits.

Commentary: Though two opinions regarding who bears financial responsibility for an aged parent appear in the Talmud, the generally accepted preference was for the parent to pay for his or her food and clothing needs. This ruling stood in conflict with an older tradition which stated that children must honor their parents by spending on them. In order to maintain harmony between the two positions, the later talmudic teachers claimed that the child's financial outlay took the form of loss of work time and the profits it might bring. The child, then, was expected to help feed and clothe the parent if that was necessary. The food and clothing, however, was paid for by the parent.

Analysis of the Text as a Whole

The talmudic text has introduced us to a number of concepts. "Respect" and "honor," for example, are not emotions for the Talmud. Rather, they are concrete acts directed toward different aspects of the parent as human being. The acts that constitute "respect" are directed toward the parent's psyche. The acts subsumed under "honor" are direct-ed to the physical needs of the parent. Thus, the emotional and physical well-being of the aged parent is the focus of talmudic concern. Mere lip service to these issues is insufficient. Feeling respectful or feeling honor is not central to the Talmud. Rather, acting in a way that makes the par-ent feel that he or she is a significant and special person to the child is what Jewish law demands. Note, the Talmud does not preclude an inter-nalized sense of respect and honor for one's parents. Indeed, it might even encourage it, but the central focus here is proper action, the most basically ethical behavior toward those who made one's life possible.

The Talmud's unwillingness to understand the Torah's commands of honor and respect as emotional is, I believe, greatly insightful. It recog-nizes that no one, not even God, can command the emotions of another. We feel what we feel. We can do little else. But appropriate and proper behavior, that is another matter. We can act as we should. It may take effort and will, but in the end we are the masters of our actions. Therefore, the realm of actions is the appropriate concern of mitzvot, commandments. To a great degree, this leaves the question of how one feels about one's parents out of the issue, and rightly so. All children feel ambivalent feelings toward their parents. How else can it be when the parent has been provider but also disciplinarian, compassionate supporter but also implacable judge? The talmudic message is, in the face of this, that if one's parents were decent parents, complicated feelings about them do not provide excuses for inappropriate responses to their needs, emotional or physical. To no less a degree that talmudic approach removes from children the burden of guilt for negative feelings about their parents. These may be inevitable, but, for Jewish law and thought, they are beside the point. In essence, what one actually does in the relationship between parent and child is ethically more significant than what one feels at any given moment.

The question "Who pays?" also leads to some consideration of the talmudic way of doing things. Clearly, the Talmud is eminently pragmatic. If it determines that honor is observed by physical support in the forms of feeding, clothing, and accompanying, then its pragmatic thinkers and contributors ask the question "Who pays for this?" They knew that ethics cannot survive without realistic programs and "game plans" for carrying them out. This, too, is part of the rabbinic genius. The Sages not only state the moral imperative, they also give some meaningful attention to the way such an imperative might be implemented.

Now to the argument over "Who pays?" itself. We note that there are two views, R. Judah's and R. Nathan b. Oshaiah's. On the face of the matter it would appear that R. Judah's view should prevail. After all, the command to honor is directed toward the child! Therefore, let the child pay for the parent's honor. Indeed, one wonders what prompted R. Nathan b. Oshaiah to propound his position. Yet, in answering a question in regard to the final decision in this case, the prevailing rabbinic view was that a parent should pay for the physical elements of his or her honor. Why?

It is here that other elements of the passage come into play. We noted above that the Talmud found in the two different verses regarding the relationship of child to parent two different modes of the relationship, the psychological and the physical. "Respect," to reiterate, demands action that allows the parent to feel specially valued and revered. "Respect" from the child is meant to encourage a sense of worth, even power, in the parent. That is why the interpretation of the *Shulchan Aruch* regarding this passage is so striking. As noted above, it understands the noninterference of the child in the disputes of the parent as the child's resisting involvement *in support of the parent's position.* One wonders why, out of respect, one would be "nonsupportive" in such a case.

The answer lies in the result. Let us say the parent wins the dispute. There will always be that nagging doubt that it was not on his or her own merit that he or she won. Rather, the "win" might be due to the child's presence or strength or intelligence. In short, the parent has to contend with the possibility that he cannot fight his own battles. It may even be true, but how does this "supported" parent feel? The parental role is to support children, fight their battles, protect and defend them. The inversion of rules has to be painful for a parent, especially if he or she is factually in need of such support. Herein lies the point of juncture between the commandments of "respect" and "honor."

Let us again picture the parent who needs to be fed, clothed, and brought in and out by another person. That is the picture of a person whose physical capabilities are now extremely limited. An adult life of self-direction and self-support is no longer possible. One's sense of dignity in such a situation is frontally attacked. One is forcibly turned back into a child, at least at the physical level. The psychic degradation can be no less than horrendous. Now the question "Who pays?" points to more than the practical details of handling the commandment of "honor." It points to the facets of self-worth, control, and decision making that are the components of independence, the very thing that the incapacitated aged lack.

Money is one of the most highly charged commodities known to humankind. It symbolizes value at more than the economic level. The talmudic world understood that when it punned about money, which is sometimes called *damim* in Hebrew. "*Damim* is a double entendre," the Sages said, because it means both money and blood. And "the blood is the life." This is not a statement that means that money is worth everything or that life is money. But it is a statement that money makes independence possible. Independence fosters a sense of self-worth, and self-worth makes life meaningful. For a child to say to a greatly diminished parent "I'll pay" when the parent still has personal assets is murderous. It kills the parental self. Here is the last framework in which the parent can be a self-directing, self-supporting person, and the child refuses to allow him or her that right and pleasure. "Who pays for accoutrements of honor?" If the mitzvah to revere one's parents means anything, then the parent pays if he or she can. This is what R. Nathan b. Oshaiah understood. This is what the Rabbis accepted as law.

But what is the child to do? The tradition demands that he or she give something tangible to the parent in order to fulfill the command to honor. Indeed the talmudic answer is succinct and powerful: more than your money, which is a mere external when all is said and done, give your time, your presence, your services. The moments taken from your own valuable time—and time, of all things, is truly life—share that with your parents if you wish to honor them. If they are not incapacitated physically, let them do for themselves, decide for themselves. They have been doing that for all their independent adult lives. Remember that it is not our role, no matter how tempting in order to finally claim our independence, to diminish our parents in the guise of "caring for" them. Here, the Talmud's lore is most to the point: There are children who feed their parents pheasant and drive them from the world-that-is. And there are children who cause their parents to grind at the millstone and grant them the world-to-come (BT *Kiddushin* 31a–b).

Spiritual and Philosophical Implications

As we have seen, the question, "Who pays?" points to a Jewish concern for human dignity and self-worth. It asks people in positions of relative strength to remember that others once had that strength and to consider what its loss means. Once having done that, Jewish ethics demands that we act in light of the recognition of how hurtful such loss is. But why this concern for dignity? Is it not enough that the aged be cared for by whatever means? Here we enter the realm of the spiritual and philosophical background that leads to the question "Who pays?"

For a moment I would like to approach the issue of Jewish concerns negatively. The stake of Judaism in the value of the individual is not predicated on the pragmatic attitude of "What have you done for me lately? What can you do for me now?" Nor is the concern prophylactic in the sense that I must behave properly toward my aged parents lest my children learn how to deal with me improperly when I am old. Rather, the Jewish message of this talmudic passage is something else. That something else is rooted in the Jewish conception of the creation of humanity in God's Image.

What do we mean when we speak of God's Image? Obviously, it does not mean "in God's form," since the Torah reminds Israel repeatedly that it saw no form when God revealed Himself/Herself at Sinai. Philosophers have sought to explain God's Image as the ability to reason. Yet, Judaism holds that mentally defective human beings are no less created in the Divine Image. That is why murdering such persons would call forth the full penalty of the law (see Genesis 9:6). No, the Image of God is more subtle. It rests in the characteristic of God that Jews proclaim twice daily as the central theological statement of Judaism: "Hear, Israel, the Eternal is our God, the Eternal is One!" That oneness is not merely unity, a thought that gained prominence only after trinitarian thinking became central to Christianity, but uniqueness. The exclamation of Israel after being saved from the Egyptians at the Sea, "Who is comparable to You among those revered as gods, Eternal God, who is like You, great in holiness?" is the finest commentary on the meaning of God's oneness and God's Image.

In light of this, when we speak of people being created in God's Image we mean that each person is absolutely unique and therefore endowed with inestimable worth. Who can replace the unique? Indeed, how can one begin to set its value? This is the core of the Jewish antipathy to counting people expressed both in Jewish lore and Jewish life. Yiddish speakers know how *"nisht eins, nisht, tzvei,"* "not one, not two," becomes a circumlocution for "one person, two people," etc. For after all is said and done, Jewish values teach us that people can be counted "one, one, one. . . ." Lowering a person's value in his or her own eyes, contributing to another's degradation in any way, these are crimes not only against the individual according to Jewish teaching, but affronts to God. Indeed, lowering oneself in one's own estimation is a failure to see oneself as what one really is: an Image of God, worth everything and worthy of everything.

What are the implications of all this for adult children and elderly parents? What is the meaning of these teachings for the care of the aged? First, the relationship of adult child to diminished parent cannot become one of inverted roles, not, at least, until it must. A parent who is old is still an adult. What life has taken away in terms of capabilities does not mean total incapacity until that state is truly reached. Whatever abilities remain that allow the aged to work, to do, to care for themselves and others must be given full rein. Any other attitude or ambience effaces the Divine Image and, thereby, destroys the life of the aged. "Who pays?" is answered by "The child" only when no choices exist. Then, knowingly, the Talmud calls the payment by its rightful name in terms of how it inevitably makes the parent feel: *tzedakah*, the closest that Hebrew can come to "charity." When choices exist, children and agencies must support independence in as many areas as possible for the aged.

Second, children are also created in God's Image. Their lives cannot be swallowed up by the crushing of their individuality under impossible burdens created by parents. Indeed, the commandments of respect and honor are incumbent upon children only when parents observe the commandments required of them. An attack upon the source of Jewish values, the Torah, by the parent invalidates the parent's rights provided by that source. Parents who have been irresponsible, cruel, neglectful, and harmful to their children have failed to uphold their obligations in Jewish law and practice to their children. Hence they have forfeited the "honor" and "respect" with which Jewish law entitles them. Yet, there are cases of unforeseen and unintended tragedy between children and aging or aged parents. The legal codes of Judaism know this and deal with such circumstances thus:

> One whose parent has become incompetent should try to deal with him/her according to his/her condition until he or she is healed. But if it is impossible for the child to bear because the parent is so radically changed, the child may go and leave the parent in the care of others.

The principle is clear. The child must do whatever is possible to carry out the requirements of "honor" and "respect" toward a decent parent. But when the parent begins to destroy the child, even in cases where the parent is not consciously doing so, the child may save himself or herself and observe the command to "honor," that is, care for the parent, by proxy. In such a case, the child "respects" the parent best by warding off the development of such hostility toward the parent that breaches of filial responsibility will become inevitable, destroying both parties' sense of worth, love, and dignity.

In conclusion, it is clear that the relationship of parents and adult children is a complicated affair. The talmudic Sages knew this to be so, hinting that "honor" and "respect" for parents had to be commanded, since they were not particularly natural responses on the part of children (BT *Kiddushin* 30b–31a). Rational use of parental prerogatives was not always gainsaid either. Hence, the Talmud placed those who struck their adult children under a ban, the equivalent of "shunning," for virtually tempting their children to sin by retaliating in kind (BT *Mo-eid Katan* 17a and Codes).

The so-called "generation gap" was not born yesterday. The intricacies of parent-child relations and appropriate and proper behavior in them were never less than complex. Because this is so, the ancient Talmud's reasonable, down-to-earth "Who pays?" and all the deep and rich spiritual background surrounding it, have much to teach us in this age of perplexed ethical and practical thinking about the aged and their care.

The Psychodynamics of
Caring for Aging Parents

RABBI DEBORAH PIPE-MAZO

As a parent of young children, I am often struck by the voluminous selection of child-rearing manuals, tomes to guide a parent through a child's first months and throughout the important formative years. These sources help parents to measure their child against a normative standard of growth and development and provide suggestions for troubleshooting. Although it is rare to find the child who meets each milestone as it is planned, most parents are comforted by the knowledge that their children seem to be on the right path, developing along what child-care experts call "a normative growth curve."

What, though, of children caring for the aging parent? Are there similar guidelines and understandings of "normalcy" by which they can gauge how a parent is faring? Is a physician able to tell an adult child what to expect on a month-to-month basis as the parent begins to fail due to old age? Sadly, the answer to these questions is no, resulting in mutual frustration, fear, and despair because of the vast unknown. Without a set path to follow, the caretaker and parent are on their own, forging into waters as yet uncharted.

Torah teaches "Honor your father and your mother that your days may be long upon the land that *Adonai* your God is giving you" (Exodus 20:12). As caretakers, we wish that every act we commit and every decision we make will translate into honor for our parents. How, then, should "honor" be understood and applied? The greatest honor we can bestow upon our parents is to live our lives in the image of the values and visions they proscribed. Thus, as we begin our journey on the paths of caretaking, it is incumbent upon us to examine the legacy that our parents bequeathed.

Yet there is an inherent disorientation with following our parents' teachings, as we are not, in turn, directing our children. Rather, we are confronting the challenges presented by a new relationship with our parents—indeed, we have to some extent become the parent and our parents, the child. We are not passing down the tradition as much as we are recycling its legacy and returning it to its source. The parent-child dynamic is flipped on its head, only to be gathered and redefined in unnatural terms.

Caretakers of aging parents, as well as the aging parents themselves, struggle most with the psychodynamics of this role reversal. The young are supposed to rely upon their elders for wisdom and counsel, and the elders are supposed to be able to provide these values and direction. It is disconcerting for everyone involved when this dynamic is turned upside down and inside out. Elders hesitate to ask for help. They feel shame and embarrassment when not able to care for themselves. Though advice and guidance from children is founded in love, the parents feel threatened and thus often cannot accept help when first offered. They fear that, by accepting help or advice from their children, their status in the family and the honor and respect due to them will change. On the other hand, children are often reticent to offer advice, lest their concern be interpreted as impudence. In addition, they feel constrained by traditional roles against taking a proactive lead, unsure of how to even begin to approach the parent in need. Thus, communication breaks down, messages are misunderstood, and in the midst of a care crisis, the family is focusing on relationships and not on the specific needs that must be addressed.

Torah can be a guide for us in this confusing and frustrating scenario. Not only are we commanded to honor our parents, we are also admonished against causing—directly or indirectly—any injury to them: "Cursed be the one who insults his father or his mother" (Deuteronomy 27:16). We insult our parents when we do not act on their behalf, in their best interest. Thus, we must openly address the discomfort and define the new relationship if we are to be successful in our new role—helping our parents to age with dignity and in comfort. Perhaps a few simple, yet firm statements are in order: "You have loved me and cared for me. Due to your guidance, I am the person I am today. Let me give back to you some of what you have taught me. Let me show you what you have shown me—that it is incumbent upon family to care for each other. Let me show you how I love you by helping you to receive the care you need."

Grieving is an essential component of caretaking. When witnessing the deterioration of a parent, it is imperative to address the emotions conjured up by these losses. Caretakers experience sadness, melancholy, feelings of being bereft and abandoned, depression, and anxiety on a regular basis. We remember and dwell upon what our parents were once able to do. We also fight against our new role and its burden, easily overwhelmed by the details and responsibility. We might relinquish our mature behaviors and act out in old, familiar patterns. Stagnancy in the past only serves as an obstacle to good care for the elder. Talk about what is happening. Keep a daily journal of feelings and thoughts. Seek help from a professional trained in grief therapy. Join a support group. Ask for help. Look into local social services. We must identify and give voice to these feelings of what it means to share in our parents' losses. It is only when we can do this that we will be able to let go of these debilitating feelings and help our parents to make safe, beneficial decisions.

Grief work, though, is not a straightforward process. As has long been documented in the annals of psychology, a caretaker will experience many stages of grief. Denial, anger, reasoning, bargaining, and acceptance are five typical stages of this process. Denial of both the process and the reality is prevalent in adult children of aging parents. We do not want to admit that our parents are failing. It is easier to make excuses for mishaps than to accept into our consciousness that new limitations are evident. Anger with an aging parent is natural, although it can become quite serious. For most of us, this anger is manifested by a thoughtless slip of the tongue or an expression of impatience. However, many aging individuals experience actual abuse by their caretakers. Needless to say, the parent, helpless to stop the hurt or neglect, suffers greatly on both a physical and psychological level.

When bargaining with God or reasoning with the doctor does not move the parent toward any noticeable progress, the caretaker shifts into acceptance of the reality of aging. Acceptance, while quite difficult, is a gift that children can give to their parents. Their ability to react and respond appropriately to their parents according to the parents' needs ensures their best possible care and a solidifying of the new parent-child relationship.

Throughout the process that leads to acceptance, patience and tolerance are important qualities for the caretaker to personify. As our parents helped to shape us into the people we are today, it is incumbent upon us to permit them to age according to their own uniqueness. This is a time when unfamiliar character traits may surface, often to the surprise or even embarrassment of adult children who thought they knew their parents well. A previously proper and well-mannered man might take to cursing his caretakers and speaking in lewd terms. Although unpleasant for everyone involved, these demonstrations provide a certain productive energy for this man. This energy helps him to bathe and clothe himself each morning. In this case, the old saying "stick with whatever works" holds great merit.

Aging parents have rights that must be respected. The highest priorities, following safety and security, are helping a parent maintain independence, preserve dignity, and retain as much control as possible. While it can be maddening to wait for a sick parent to call a doctor or become concerned enough about a certain symptom, the caretaker must respect the elder's sense of time and immediacy. Although it is not easy to stand by and permit someone we love to follow "the hard way," if a parent can do it—leave it alone. Even though you might be able to do it better or quicker, with greater finesse or aplomb, more is gained by their effort at independence than merely accomplishing a task. Maintaining their pride, preserving dignity, and reinforcing their self-image as a contributing member of society all help an elder to feel fulfillment in the midst of the aging process. When children help their parents to meet these goals and live according to their rights, the newness of the upside-down relationship quickly fades into mutual respect and acceptance. As caretakers, part of our job must be to celebrate and encourage our parents' choices and independence. In Deuteronomy 30:19, God commands us, "Choose life!" so that we might experience blessing and peace. Our parents will make choices about life and living—according to who they are, their uniqueness and character, their life experience and needs—and from these choices, because they made them, blessing and peace will be theirs.

Another source of blessing for our parents is to help them focus on what they *can* do and what they can do *well*. Help them to rediscover an old hobby or to claim an expertise. Invite them to work or school to impart to future generations what they have learned about life. Share aloud the good memories and help to re-create them in the present. Although the day-to-day relationship between caretaker and parent changes due to needs and circumstances, the psychospiritual dynamic remains the same. You are the child, the child of this parent. Seek opportunities in which that relationship can still be affirmed. Continue to ask for advice and guidance. Ask them to share stories from long ago. Include them in the daily happenings of your life. Let them know that they are significant and that you need them. The more our parents feel comfortable with us in a relationship that has been in place since the day we were born, the less they will resent and rebel against that which is new and unfamiliar.

In closing, a prayer: May the months and years ahead provide an opportunity to celebrate each child and each parent. May our experiences as both parents and children help guide us toward mutual respect, affirmation, and acceptance. May we, as caretakers, help to bring out the beauty and dignity of our aging parents, as we seek to care for them within the legacy they bestowed upon us. May we continue to grow as children, even as we parent those who gave us life.

Becoming an Expert on the Individual, Not the Disease

⌘

Kathryn Kahn

I have traveled a distance on this path since I first admitted to myself that my mother did indeed have Alzheimer's disease. In the beginning I became very skilled at denial—this disease didn't run in our family, my mother was only occasionally forgetful, she wasn't roaming the streets and hallucinating. This absolutely could not be the disease I had heard so many horrible stories about. I will never forget the day I typed "Alzheimer's" and then clicked on Search at my computer. I was all alone because I wanted no one to know that this A-word had anything to do with my mother. I hid it from my daughters as long as I could, fearing the news would change forever the way they felt toward their grandmother.

Even the close and loving relationship I had with my mother-in-law was temporarily affected. I grew distant from her. She is a vital and strong woman with all her faculties intact, and I hated her for it. Anger was a large part of my response—someone or something should pay for this dreadful card that fate dealt my mother.

I have discovered that although feelings of anger and

despair are understandable initial responses to this disease, they are probably the least helpful to the patient and the caregiver. Despair comes with shock of diagnosis when all the nightmare scenarios are explored and anticipated. It is irrelevant to the care and love that are necessary for the long term. And this *is* a long-term experience, with plenty of time to learn and become an "expert" at caring for and interacting with the person you love. It is also a chance to realize how many opportunities there are for love, laughter, and bonding in the years ahead. It is truly possible to continue a close, positive relationship on many levels—there have been wonderful times and precious memories created in spite of and in defiance of the shadow this illness has cast.

I am no authority on Alzheimer's as a disease that afflicts other people in general. I am slowly becoming knowledgeable about the way this disease has affected my mother, and, in turn, my family and myself.

These are some of the things I've learned:

- If I approach my mother with love and patience, she will respond positively and lovingly. If I approach her with anger or anxiety, she will reflect those emotions back at me. She can read my mood immediately and accurately if I allow it to affect the way I speak or behave.
- If I am abrupt and in a hurry, she will react by slowing down and resisting.
- There are times when she is again my mother in the fullest and completest sense of the word. During those periods, I can tell her my troubles, and she becomes my adviser and supporter—that this is still sometimes possible, even at this stage, is a real, if unexpected blessing.

The benefit for my mother is that I am allowing her to be needed again—to give support and comfort instead of just receiving it.

- When she becomes anxious, she often mentally retreats to an earlier (maybe safer?) time. During those periods, she thinks that I am her mother or her sister and refers to her husband as her father.

- I have learned not to waste time keeping score—evaluating who does more for my mother, especially my father, siblings, and other family members. This is a sensitive issue, and I fear that the defensiveness that guilt brings could drive a wedge between us all. I will not risk alienating a family member, perhaps forever, over my perception of who is doing "enough" for my mother.

- It is important to remind myself that my anger, toward my mother, toward myself and others, is strongest when I am most afraid.

Today I think I cracked the code of two phrases that she uses so often. The first one, "What comes next? What are we supposed to do now?" means she is feeling anxious and needing reassurance. I know that I am trying to find answers to those two important questions as well. The second is her use of the word "real." "You look so *real*" is the highest compliment my mother can pay anyone. A face that looks real offers a lifeline of meaning for her.

Today we sang the entire score of *South Pacific* and laughed through it all.

Today my mother and I pulled into the driveway of the house she's lived in for forty-five years. She turned to me and said, "Have we been here before?"

Today my mother gently corrected my sloppy grammar twice and then, with a chuckle, reminded me that as my mother, that was her job.

Today, like many days, was full of joy and despair and wonder.

Loss

"Job said in reply:
Today again my complaint is bitter;
My strength is spent on account of my groaning.
Would that I knew how to reach Him,
How to get to His dwelling-place.
I would set out my case before Him."   Job 23:1–4

Adonai, I do not know what to pray for or how to pray . . .
Even the *Mi Shebeirach* is too bright for me.
This is the long *Kaddish.* This is the darkening road.
My mother is losing her memory . . . I don't know how to get
   it back for her.

Will you consider in the balance of her fate, how she nursed
   so many,
So tenderly?
That she eased the journey of thousands through illness . . .
   faithful care,
Even until death.
That she championed the weak and the young and the lost
Every day of her life.
That she made a home that was an unfailing refuge for my
   heart . . .
That was a gallery for my small triumphs.
How everything that is good and compassionate in me is
   only the faintest echo

Of what I see in her?

Will you remember that her faith in You has always been
unshakable?

How diminished Your song of praise will be if she forgets
who You are . . .

if she forgets who i am . . .

How can this be borne?

She holds on to us, and to who she is, as tightly as she can,

But her grasp is not strong and I feel her slipping away.

Why are my hands so weak, so helpless to draw her back?

She knows this . . . she is frightened . . . she is ashamed.

The shame is mine . . .

All my life, her strength was there for me...never failing in
the face of

My despair.

What kind of child am I, who stands so useless before her
need?

How do I help her, protect her, raise her high, carry her,

Clear these dark, sticky tangles from her mind?

Keep my cries of despair silent . . . keep my love for her shin-
ing on her dimming path . . .

Will You not show some small mercy?

Is there some price I can pay for her sake?

"See, I am of small worth; what can I answer You?
I clap my hand to my mouth.
I have spoken once, and will not reply;
Twice, and will do so no more."   Job 40:4–5

Honor Your Father and Mother:
Caregiving as a Halachic Responsiblity

RABBI RUTH LANGER

A striking feature of the rabbinic discussions of this mitzvah is the absence of a pronouncement specific to young children's relationships with their parents and, conversely, the relatively detailed attention to situations that pertain more readily to adult children and their elders. We never outgrow the obligation to honor our parents; indeed, the obligation grows more significant as we and our parents age.[1]

The halachic tradition recognizes that one of the most intense and difficult phases of the child-parent relationship is often toward the end of the parent's life. Age generates physical and mental debilities that create dependency, often accompanied by personality changes that threaten to undermine the familial relationship. But the rabbinic discussions took place at a time when reaching old age at all was rare, and extended chronic illness was relatively uncommon. In our day, when medical advances and longer life spans have dramatically increased the likelihood that any individual parent will spend an extended period in frail physical and mental health, the question of the halachically required nuances of "honoring one's parents" needs to be reopened with much deeper attention paid to the repercussions of several aspects of the changed reality of our times.

Dedicated to the memory of Marcus Lester and Maxine Goldmark Aaron, and in honor of their children, who honored, revered, and loved them.

Reprinted, with changes, from Jacob, Walter and Moshe Zemer, eds. *Aging and the Aged in Jewish Law: Essays and Responsa*. Pittsburgh and Tel Aviv: Freehof Institute of Progressive Halakhah, 1998, 22–41.

By juxtaposing the halachic tradition and the results of contemporary gerontological research, we can reach new and deeper understandings of the halachic tradition. These understandings can then help us formulate a late twentieth-century statement about filial obligations to parents that is sensitive both to the beauties of the Jewish legal-ethical tradition and to the realities of modern life.

We must begin with a review of the halachic sources. The source of the mitzvah lies, of course, in the fifth of the Ten Commandments, which rules, "Honor you father and mother. . . " and in Leviticus 19:3, which says, "Each person shall revere (or fear) his mother and father." The earliest midrashic collections juxtapose these verses with similar ones demanding honor and reverence of God to answer the critical question: precisely how does one fulfill this mitzvah, known as *kibud av va-eim*, honoring father and mother?[2] In the Ten Commandments father precedes mother, whereas in Leviticus the order is reversed. Midrash by definition finds this meaningful and suggests that this reversed order indicates that, in observing this commandment, children may not privilege one parent over the other: both are equal.

The Ten Commandments and Leviticus also use two different verbs, "honor" and "revere." These two verbs also appear in connection with commanded human relationships with God. This not only lends extreme gravity to the commanded relationship with parents, placing it among those commandments that have "no measure,"[3] but also allows the Rabbis to develop the details of this relationship by giving greater indication of their practical meaning. Proverbs 3:9 reads, "Honor God with your wealth." Honoring, then, is expressed materially; to honor parents refers to the provision of goods and, even more importantly, of services. The tannaitic tradition establishes that dutiful children express honor by ensuring food and drink, clothing and shelter, and by accompanying parents as they enter and leave. In other words, children have an obligation to tend to their parents' needs. A question we shall need to confront later is whether this demands direct caregiving or just indicates the provision of care.

Here the rabbinic traditions specifically indicate that the parent should pay for the substance of this care; and if the parent is destitute, any contribution from the child falls in the category of *tzedakah*, where in any case provision for one's own family takes priority. The implication of removing the financial element from the commandment to honor parents is primarily that children are not required to impoverish themselves to maintain their parents' accustomed standard of living.[4]

Showing reverence to parents is also analogous to showing reverence to God and, even more directly, to showing reverence to a sage or teacher. The Rabbis indicate that this means respecting parents' social space, neither standing nor sitting in their accustomed spots and respecting their authority and dignity, neither contradicting them nor inserting oneself into their decisions. An outward symbol of this respect is always to refer to parents by an appropriate title and not by their given names. As Gerald Blidstein writes in his comprehensive book on this commandment, "The principle behind this pattern is clear: nothing is to be done that might diminish the dignity, and hence the feeling of worth, of one's parents."[5]

Although these details are important and give substance and shape to the commandments, a few overarching points deserve special emphasis. Maimonides begins his discussion of our issue saying, "Honoring parents is an *important* positive commandment."[6] It is not merely ethically, socially, or naturally important; rather, the Torah's implied equation of relationships with parents and relationships with God elevates the mitzvah of honoring parents. Like every social relationship, but even more so, its implications are not solely in the human realm, but reflect primarily on one's fealty and obedience to God's command. Fulfillment of this commandment comes primarily, therefore, within the rabbinic system, out of an absolute obligation originating in God. The specifics of children's relationships with their parents, whether there is a bond of love or of social obligation based on services received from parents, is essentially irrelevant. Love and prior relationships are indeed a reason for honoring one's parents, but their absence by no means exempts children from the obligation to fulfill the commandment; fulfilling the commandment solely on the basis of love or personal human obligation does not raise it to its highest spiritual level.[7]

We need to place this observation in conversation with the prevailing discussions in the gerontological literature on caregiving relationships. A 1993 Gallup poll indicated that 85 percent of Americans consider it the responsibility of adult children to care for their parents.[8] Some have tried to claim that this pervasive sense of filial obligation is based on understandings of an economic exchange of services.[9] Just as parents cared for children in their youth, so, now, children have an obligation to pay the debt and return the favor. Social scientists, however, recognize that this model is insufficient. The parent who cares for a healthy child makes an investment in the future and looks forward to the satisfaction of watching that child become a contributing member of society. The motivation for providing that care is not commonly, in our twentieth-century American world, a conscious investment in establishing a care situation for one's own old age.[10] In contrast, the child that cares for an aged parent cannot realistically expect a rosy future. Thus, although from the parent's perspective there may be an element of exchange, from the child's perspective, the emotional and psychological burden of the caregiving is substantially different.[11]

Jewish tradition, from the Bible on, presents a model for this relationship that at first glance seems to be equivalent to this exchange theory; but the majority of discussions speak of filial piety not as an exchange of services, but rather as an expression of gratitude, an ethical rather than an economic category. Especially because of God's involvement in everything the child should be grateful for—life, nurturing, and so forth— ingratitude to parents is seen as leading to or even as an actual expression of ingratitude to God and a denigration or denial of God's historical and covenental relationship with Israel.[12] Children do not merely repay their parents for services rendered to them in their childhood; rather, they act on the basis of an interpersonal relationship that is a microcosm of their relationship with God.

This would seem to bring us closer to an alternative social science model, one that derives from a twentieth-century understanding of interpersonal behavior. This model suggests that the sense of filial obligation to parents arises, and should be understood as arising, from the love and friendship that has developed between the generations. Nothing is "owed" that must be returned, but the social relationship itself generates the caregiving.[13] Because of this relationship, because of a desire to meet the deepest needs of the loved one, the caregiver renders care. On the other hand, a neutral or negative social relationship will not create a caregiving situation. Thus, in this model, estranged children have no filial obligation at all, and, in addition, the stresses on the caregiver and the caregiver's family of providing long-term care, of which we will speak more later, could easily erode such a relationship, making the basis for provision of care shaky at best.

In spite of its obvious problems, this model does influence our world. Tamara K. Hareven suggests that the source of the growing sense of isolation of the elderly in contemporary society stems from exactly this shift in common views of the family, from an "instrumental" one of shared obligations to one that understands "sentimentality and intimacy" to be the forces holding the family together.[14] It follows, then, that the sentimental element of a parent-child relationship does not enter into the halachic determinations of the child's responsibilities. Indeed, Jewish law explicitly acknowledges the difficulties and stresses of the parent-child relationship, both under "normal" circumstances and as exacerbated in situations of ill health.[15] It is exactly these challenges to the filial relationship that drive the halachic system to elevate the commandment to honor parents to such an absolute, insisting that children's honor and respect for their parents must be as unconditional as their relationship with God. The gratitude expressed in filial piety is not a matter of exchange or of love on the earthly level. The emotional health of the parent-child relationship is secondary at best. Responsibility and obligation take precedence and ensure that the needs of the elderly are appropriately met.[16]

Having established the absolute and elevated nature of the filial obligation to honor and respect parents, we need now consider some details of the relationship and, particularly, to ask if it has limits, too. Significant contemporary research on caregiving families looks to understand, measure, and alleviate the stress created when a family must bring into its midst or take responsibility for a now physically or mentally debilitated parent. Although having a dependent, elderly parent has become a normative experience, it is one that exceeds the capacities of many families to cope. This can be attributed to many factors, most significantly demographic shifts: there are more elderly because people are living longer, but there are fewer caregivers because of declining birth rates. This has increased the odds that children will need to become caregivers and that the caregivers themselves will be older. In addition, death now more often follows chronic, long-term illness, increasing the time span for which caregiving is required. Consequently, "adult children provide more care and more difficult care to more parents over much longer periods of time than they did in the good old days."[17]

Elaine Brody documents the direct effects of this caregiving situation on the caregiver herself (the vast majority of American caregivers are wives, daughters, and daughters-in-law). These include financial hardship, a decline in her own health, mental health symptoms from restrictions on her own time and freedom, isolation, conflicting demands from competing responsibilities, and interference with her lifestyle and recreational activities. These pressures can reactivate latent problems in the child's relationship with her parent and with the rest of her family, creating instability in the home in general. Brody and many others considering this sort of data seriously criticize the trend in American public policy that, although insisting that children continue to be the primary caregivers for their elderly parents, pays insufficient attention to ensuring that support systems are available, of desirable quality, and known to the caregivers before they reach a point of utter crisis. Study after study shows the value to the elderly of family care. The question is whether the family can be equipped to meet the demands created in today's world.

The rabbinic discussions on this issue were obviously written before the modern demographic shift that so changed the incidence of caregiving. In light of this, it is surprising how little contemporary discussion there is of questions of filial responsibility for extended caregiving, especially in cases like Alzheimer's disease, where the personality changes are so marked, or even in less severe situations where the normal, nonpathological intensification of personality traits in old age can reactivate the childhood love-hate relationship with the parent, making operation under the rabbinic guidelines for honor and reverence difficult. Most modern authorities simply assume that the halachah developed for short-term caregiving applies directly and obviously to contemporary demographics.[18] The parameters set out by the traditional rabbinic discussions are clear. Even if the parent is mentally disabled to an extent that causes the child distress, the child must assiduously preserve a stance of reverence of honor to the parent. In Maimonides' classic recapitulation of the talmudic teachings, he writes:

> What is the extent of honoring one's father and mother? Even
> if they took his pouch of gold coins and, in his presence, threw
> it into the sea, he should not reproach them or show distress
> or anger in their presence, but rather he should accept the
> decree of Scripture [God] and be silent.

What is the extent of revering them? Even if one were wearing expensive clothing, sitting at the head of an assembly, and one's parents came, tore his clothes, hit him on the head, and spit in his face, he should not reproach them. Instead, he should be silent and have reverence and fear of the King, the King of kings, who has commanded him thus [to revere his parents].

For even if a king of flesh and blood had decreed something that hurt him more than this, he could not struggle against it; so how much more so [is this] the case regarding the decree of the One who spoke and the world came to be according to His will?[19]

Typically, the talmudic tradition that Maimonides summarizes here deals with the extreme situation. What could most easily and seemingly legitimately lead the most dutiful, reverent children to abandon their proper filial behavior? Obviously, irrational, destructive, humiliating behavior by their parents, indicating their own lack of respect for the children.

To highlight the abnormality of these situations, Maimonides juxtaposes with this the legal tradition that parents are under obligation to make it possible for their children to fulfill their obligations to show honor and reverence. Parents should not only avoid unreasonable demands, but should even go out of their way explicitly to forego some of the honor due them so as not to cause the children to stumble.[20] In the extreme case of the parent who strikes a grown child, a court may excommunicate that parent, because this action makes the child's ability to respond within the parameters of honoring and revering almost impossible.[21] The halachah actively discourages and condemns such extreme abuse of parental rights, to the point of expelling the abusive parent from the community—in many ways the most serious punishment available to the medieval rabbinic courts. Yet, the halachah also maintains the child's obligations to honor and revere as absolute.

Under normal, healthy circumstances, therefore, a parent should never literally throw away the child's money or publicly severely humiliate the grown child. Indeed, most commentators understand the parents in these rabbinic examples to be medically out of control, most likely mentally ill or senile. In such a case, although the children's halachic obligations toward their parents may and must be stretched to the limit of endurance, the parents themselves are not considered responsible for their actions. A senile parent is not excommunicated, God forbid! Rather, however difficult, the child must compassionately continue to show utmost reverence and honor. Why? Not only because of the intrinsic nature of the relationship, but also because the way that one behaves toward one's parents reflects on one's relationship with God. Given all this, the difficult question must be raised: Is there a point where the debilitation of the parent, primarily mental but also physical, might create a situation of such conflict that the ideal of children's personal service to parents must be given up in deference to maintaining a greater attitude of honor and reverence?[22] Indeed, this is Maimonides' understanding of the story relayed in the Talmud about the Babylonian Rav Assi. The Talmud tells us:

> Rav Assi had an elderly mother. She said to him, "I want jewelry." He provided it for her. "I want a husband." [He replied,] "I'll search for one for you." "I want a husband who will be as handsome as you." He left her and went to the Land of Israel. He heard that she was following after him, so he went to Rabbi Yochanan and asked him, "Is it permissible to leave the Land of Israel?" [Rabbi Yochanan] replied, "It is forbidden." Rav Assi [continued,] "What if I am going to meet my mother?" He replied, "I do not know." Rav Assi waited a bit, and then went back again. [Rav Yochanan] said to him, "Assi, you have decided that you want to go. May God let you return in peace."
>
> Rav Assi went to Rabbi Elazar and said to him, "God forbid, is Rabbi Yochanan angry with me?" Rabbi Elazar asked, "What did he say to you?" He replied, "May God let you return in peace." Rabbi Elazar replied, "If he were angry, he would not have blessed you."
>
> In the meantime, he heard that it was his mother's coffin that was coming. He said, "If I had known, I wouldn't have had to leave."[23]

There are levels of complexity to this story with which we do not have to deal here. Several points are clear. The Babylonian Rav Assi is torn between two competing halachically important obligations—showing proper honor and reverence to his mother and dwelling in the Land of Israel. His mother, by her demands, drives him to the point that remaining in her presence is impossible, enabling him to give priority to the obligation to live in Israel. His ambivalence about this ranking is evident in his dithering over whether it is proper to leave the land to go to meet his mother on her journey to be again with him. It is also extremely important as an insight into the conflicts felt by any dutiful child who chooses, even of necessity, to leave behind an elderly parent.

Critical to our discussion, here, is the clear statement of the Talmud that what drove Rav Assi to leave were the unreasonable and unfulfillable demands that his mother was placing on him.[24] As a dutiful son, Rav Assi could not outright refuse her unreasonable demands; he did provide jewelry and said he would look into finding her a husband, but when the badgering turned to unreasonable specifics about that husband, that he be handsome and, we assume, youthful, like Rav Assi himself, were polite, ambiguous answers possible? The primary interpretative tradition of this passage was developed by Maimonides. He places Rav Assi's mother in the same category as the parent who throws away the child's money or embarrasses the adult child but who must be treated compassionately. But even this has its limits. Maimonides writes:

> One whose father or mother has become mentally impaired should try to treat them according to their mental ability with pity for them. But if he cannot stand it, because they have become too deranged, he should leave them and go, directing others to treat them appropriately.[25]

Maimonides' interpretation, with which not all sages agreed, but which became mainstream halachah, particularly with Joseph Caro's explicit acceptance of it in his *Beit Yosef* and *Shulchan Aruch*,[26] is that filial obligations to honor and revere parents are an absolute that must be upheld under the most difficult of circumstances. Yet, because Rav Assi is not criticized for leaving his mother, this must be seen as a precedent. He did try to honor her wishes, but she pushed him too far. When that point is reached, it is perfectly appropriate, according to Jewish law, for the child to leave the parent so that the relationship will not deteriorate and the child will not be forced into actions lacking honor and reverence. Maimonides adds a significant point. The child is not free simply to abandon the parent. Rather, the child must specifically delegate the care of the parent to others. In arranging this care, the child's serious responsibility is to ensure that these others will treat the debilitated parent appropriately.

Turning to a nursing home placement, in-home nursing services, or some part-time arrangement that relieves the child of fulltime caregiving is thus fully appropriate under Jewish law when the child's attempts to provide care will result only in a deterioration of the relationship, causing the child to manifest a lack of honor or reverence to the parent. The point at which this occurs will obviously vary from case to case, and each decision must be reached individually. There are some important issues, however, in which halachah can and should inform our choices.[27]

1. We live in a society that places high value on independence and does not consider multigenerational living arrangements the norm. Children should consider seriously the impact on the parents' sense of dignity and self-worth if parents are forced to take up residence in a child's home. If parents and children are not already living in close proximity, it may well unduly undermine the parents' independence to be asked to move and be uprooted from their existing social network. If the parents deeply value independence, the choice of an assisted living facility or nursing care in the parents' home, if affordable and medically appropriate, may be the best way to demonstrate reverence for the dignity and sense of self-worth of the parents.

2. Certain cases clearly suggest third-party care. When physical modesty, particularly concerning bodily functions and hygiene, have been characteristics of the relationship between parent and child, calling on the child to bathe the parent and manage incontinence may be inappropriate.

Even if the parent is no longer aware of the loss of dignity involved, the child has an obligation to treat the parent as if his or her dignity is intact. Such care may be better delegated to an unrelated third party.

3. This is all the more true in cases where the senile parent requires physical restraint,[28] strictness in discipline, or painful treatment.

Although such painful measures may be medically fully necessary and justifiable, they nevertheless undermine the parent's dignity, which the child is required to respect at all cost.

4. Once children decide to delegate care to someone else, certain considerations generated by the children's mandate to honor and revere their parents ought to guide their selections of substitute caregivers. Various contemporary rabbis suggest that children ensure that these caregivers be ones who will respect the dignity of the parents as much as possible. Attention should be paid particularly to matters Jewish tradition identifies as signifying honor and respect. Caregivers should address the parents by the titles to which they have been accustomed and not infantilize them by automatically using their first names. Caregivers should be professionals who know and can implement emerging technologies that maximize the parents' abilities to be independent. In addition, the parents should be allowed and encouraged to continue in whatever decision-making capacities are possible. All attempts must be taken not to diminish the parents' adulthood and sense of self-worth.

5. When parents must be removed from their own homes, a personal space should be re-created for them in their new settings. Not only should they be able to surround themselves with treasured and familiar possessions, but also, ideally, they should not be placed in programs requiring their participation in activities that have never been of value to them. Those who have filled their lives with intellectual pursuits ought to have an outlet by which to continue them to the extent of their abilities and not be pushed into a day camp roster of crafts, music, and games. Similarly, those who have been Jewishly involved ought to be in a setting that encourages and deepens this commitment.

6. Traditional halachah exempts married women from all responsibility toward their parents from an assumption that their responsibilities to their husbands take priority. Consequently, it expects sons to bear the primary responsibility for ensuring appropriate care for their parents and actively demonstrating honor and reverence.[29] We may be uncomfortable with this definition of gender roles, particularly since we cannot shrug aside its obvious conflict with the reality that, in America today, the vast majority of caregiving children are women, daughters, and daughters-in-law, even among women who have otherwise broken from traditional gender stereotypes in their lives.[30] This is an area of conventional

women's concern in which Judaism fully supports an equalization or shifting of the burden.[31]

7. A final and difficult issue. The rabbinic discussions assume a basic flexibility in the children's employment situations. Although the provisions for the parents' care come, if possible, from the parents' own financial resources, the halachah is explicit that the service aspects of the care must be rendered in person, and it is only the children's emotional and physical inability to care properly for their parents within the parameters of honor and reverence that can exempt the children from this personal duty. Financial hardships caused by time taken from work are not justifiable reasons for delegating one's caregiving responsibilities.[32] Indeed, in a substantial percentage of caregiving families, women have cut back on or given up employment to care for parents.

To begin with, we must ask to what extent this actually does conflict with contemporary American expectations. As Elaine Brody has demonstrated, although over the last generation or two, many women have entered the work place motivated more by financial necessity than by issues of personal satisfaction, 28 percent of the nonworking female caregivers in her study had given up their jobs to care for parents, and a similar number of working women were considering doing so or at least cutting back their hours.[33] In essence, then, American families, or women, at least, often do conform with the halachic requirement of placing parental care over issues of income.

The challenge remains to find some halachically acceptable alternatives for cases where it is neither desirable nor feasible for the children to rearrange their work responsibilities to care for parents. Some possible paths to a solution might be:

1. When parents are not totally debilitated mentally, they have the obligation to lessen the demands made on their children for personal service. The halachic tradition encourages the parent to be *moheil al k'vodo*, to release children from some of the stiffer requirements of expressing honor and reverence. Parents sensitized in younger years to these issues may well be encouraged to discuss the eventuality of their loss of independence and to state a preference for third-party care, should it become necessary.[34]

2. Greater attention to concerns for parental modesty and independence may make personal caregiving by children less desirable. If the child is not providing full-time care, employment may not need to be sacrificed.

3. One might further question whether full-time personal parental caregiving is the only way to demonstrate proper honor. If parents can delegate child-rearing tasks to nannies and day-care centers, should they not also be legitimately able to rely on part-time caregivers for elderly parents? Study after study demonstrates that the parent-child relationship is not harmed when a child receives care in a quality setting staffed with professionally trained teachers; my personal experience shows that the child's life can be significantly enhanced. The same may well be true for debilitated parents. They may indeed benefit from third-party care by those who are trained to provide appropriate stimulation of both the body and the mind. If this is the case, then the provision of third-party care, which incidentally allows the child to work, can actually be a mode of personal service, of demonstrating honor and reverence.

These are issues that affect not only individual children with elderly parents, but the community as a whole and its public policy. Where civil government decisions rely on the research of gerontologists for guidance, the Jewish community has an additional source, the traditions of halachah. Although on the one hand, the halachic tradition portrays filial caregiving as an absolute requirement, it does create an outlet for the stresses involved in the parent-child relationship. First of all, the tradition tries to shift the caregiving from an earth-bound burden to a positive statement of a relationship with God, with a God who could not have the debilitations and irritating personality quirks of one's debilitated parent. The onerous care thus becomes not a depressing burden of watching the decline and anticipating the ultimate loss of a parent; it becomes an expression of an enduring positive relationship with the Divine. Whether this actually helps alleviate the stresses of caring for a parent obviously depends on the piety or the potential for piety of the child, but it is a road to contemplate and teach.

Secondly, unlike popular American values, Jewish tradition does not absolutely require personal care under all circumstances; rather, it legitimatizes third-party care when appropriate personal care is no longer possible or adequate. Thus, although the decision to place a parent in a nursing home or some other program or facility can never be easy, Judaism does teach that there are times when it is fully appropriate and should not be approached with a sense of guilt. The community thus has a responsibility to ensure the availability of quality facilities and to make financial resources available to those who require aid.

Finally, the halachah establishes guidelines that help ensure the highest level of third-party care, enabling parents to end their lives with maximum dignity and self-esteem. Thus, while acknowledging that caring for aged parents is never easy, the halachah approaches the situation realistically and helps the caregivers rise above the necessary stress of the situation.

The Gift of a Lifetime

cҽ ℬↄ

Laura Sperling

The phone rang Thursday at 2 P.M. on a sunny July afternoon. The dreaded call, regarding the results of Mom's exploratory surgery, came two hours earlier than I had expected. Her pancreatic cancer had spread to the stomach and liver. There was nothing to be done except deal with it.

It's a long way from Bainbridge Island, Washington, to Los Angeles, California, in more ways than one. What to do? Dad was not in good health; Mom's prognosis was a rather grim three- to six-month life expectancy of pain, starvation, and extreme suffering. A decision had to be made. My husband looked into my eyes and, with tears in his, said, "You've got to go down to LA to take care of your mother and your father for as long as it takes, or you won't be able to feel any peace at your mother's funeral." I didn't fully comprehend it at the time, but this was my first gift.

Our children were relatively independent. Our daughter, Margit, was soon to move into her dorm, as a freshman at the University of Washington. Our son, Eli, was ready to begin his freshman year in high school. My husband, Scott, was the associate rabbi at a large synagogue in the Northwest. He is my best friend and pillar of support and strength. His life is always consumed by work. As a working musician, music teacher, and recording artist, I am used to tap dancing at many parties. My mother's dire situation, our family's love, and my sense of obligation spoke to me, and I was gone.

Finding myself sleeping and practicing flute in my old bedroom and driving my mother's car was indeed very strange. Looking out the bedroom window to mature fuchsia-colored ice plant flowers once more became a familiar comfort. No towering cedar and Douglas fir to keep me company. I was, once more, living at home with my parents—after twenty-five years. I was still feeling like the daughter, yet here I was, establishing and running an intensive medical operation for mom. Now, taking care of the house, planning and cooking meals, constant doctor and hospital visits, phone calls and insurance nightmares, these were my new job. I became trained to be my mother's nurse, business manager, and aggressive advocate. I administered every manner of medication, including intravenous hydrations and medicines. Yet, despite the long hours and complex challenges, the ability to be there for my parents, especially for my mother, over a continuous period of time was a profound sacrifice and gift that I could give her. She certainly would have done this for me.

I found myself constantly inventing my next task. I would ask myself, "How can I make her more comfortable?" I'd invite her to spend as much time as possible in our beautiful garden and take barefoot walks on the cool grass. We'd investigate each flower; smelling fresh rose blooms and elegant lilies. She'd receive great relief when I'd massage her feet and back. Her spirits were buoyed by sitting outdoors, under moonlit skies, chatting with neighbors.

I knew that sooner or later we would have what I referred to as the "ultimate conversations." These talks, about life and death, spirit and destiny, unfairness, pain, anger and loss, were another gift . . . for both of us. Taking cues from Mom, looking deeply into her frightened eyes, being as tender and smart as she, I reciprocated the love she had always given me.

Our daughter, Margit, spent two weeks with her grandparents and me before the semester began. From the very start, she was in the trenches with me. Her precious time with her beloved grandma created a bond that went beyond words. Other than those two weeks with Margit, I didn't see my family until the funeral. During these months, long-distance calls to family and friends were my lifeline.

After hospice skillfully guided us through our most difficult passage, I knew I had to pack up and sell my parents' home of forty-five years. I felt that I had only one choice for caring for my dad. From the very beginning, it was clear to me that he was my second patient. Many among our extended family were aging and infirm, my brother lives in Hawaii, and for me, then, there was only one choice. Dad would be on Bainbridge Island, and we would have another huge chapter ahead of us.

Unfortunately, as a result of my father's intense depression, broken heart, and declining physical and mental condition, the assisted living center on the island became, after only five weeks, inappropriate for his needs. Again, we were faced with the agonizing question of what to do for Dad.

A long, rich life as synagogue members, having Jewish friends, and being lovers of Jewish music represented our comforts and roots. This connection has been crucially important throughout our lives, and especially now in this final phase of Dad's life. Despite the long distance between our home and Seattle's Seward Park neighborhood, the rich Jewish atmosphere of the Kline Galland Home made it the obvious choice for Dad's new home.

Every part of his life had turned inside out, and he was in total confusion, as evidenced by the rapid onset of his dementia. He had become another one of my children. I was still conducting a large-scale operation, coordinating a confusing maze of insurance, legal, and financial issues. Now, I was his full-time advocate and manager. At least I was in my own home.

My new extended family has become the friends and new surrogate aunts and uncles of the Kline Galland Home. I can now extend my gifts of music, love, and caring to them, along with my father. When I perform there, in front of my father, I am struck by this tough new reality we both face. Our new life has brought many changes. I sat in the nursing home's huge dining room for Passover seder, rather than in my own home. I danced with my father at the gala New Year's ball, guiding his halting and unsure steps, just as he had guided me on the dance floor when I was a little girl. I was now taking him on picnic dinners by the shores of the lake, reflections of many happy moments from my childhood.

Each visit to my father requires a thirty-five minute ferryboat commute and a long freeway drive both coming and going. This often means ample time for anxiety to build before a visit and long, quiet times for reflection after a visit. I have time to consider how life's rules are not necessarily enforced with fairness. Yet, I also want to believe that it is true that we get back what we give in life. I have discovered that the gifts and the pains of growing up; the constant acquisition of self-knowledge are as poignant for me now as they are for my children at their tender ages. But more than anything else I have come to know that the love of family is truly the gift of a lifetime.

ᏩᎻᎻᏁᎧ

A Jewish Way of Thinking
about Nursing Homes

RABBI SHELDON MARDER

How good and how pleasant it is
that brothers dwell together.
It is like fine oil on the head
running down onto the beard,
the beard of Aaron,
that comes down over the collar of his robe;
like the dew of Hermon
that falls upon the mountains of Zion.
There Adonai *ordained blessing,*
everlasting life.

Psalm 133

The author of Psalm 133 thought a great deal about the source of goodness in our lives. The psalm's moist images—oil and dew—are metaphors of abundance: rich oil flowing down Aaron's body, refreshing dew flowing from mountaintop to parched land below. God's blessings are abundant.

Psalm 133 is also a praise of family unity: it is good and pleasant when we dwell together. Indeed, the Psalmist's message is this: when we dwell together, God's blessing of everlasting life flows into our lives.[1] But this buoyant view of life also suggests profound questions for families wrestling with the crises of aging—especially nursing home placement. Is it possible to preserve family unity when we *cannot* dwell together? Are God's blessings still ours when the prospect of nursing home placement erects emotional as well as physical walls between us and those we love? As one of the secular self-help guides puts it:

> You hoped it would never happen. Maybe you even promised yourself or your parent it would never happen. But at some point—perhaps after great effort to avoid it, disputes with siblings and agonizing days of sadness and indecision—it becomes clear that moving your parent into a nursing home is the only practical thing to do.[2]

From a Jewish perspective, however, is it the right thing to do? Families face a "health-care delivery system" that can alienate parents, children, and siblings from one another and erode an older person's sense of self-worth and peace of mind. Thus, in our thinking about nursing home placement, we realize that what we need is something Medicare, Medicaid, and self-help books were never meant to provide: *reservoirs of faith and tradition* to nourish our spirit during life's most difficult passages. And so we turn to our people's source of faith and tradition; we turn to Torah.

> *Honor your father and your mother. . . .*
>
> Exodus 20:12

> *Each person shall revere his mother and his father.*
>
> Leviticus 19:3

"We never outgrow the obligation to honor our parents," writes Rabbi Ruth Langer. In fact, she argues, this obligation becomes ever more critical as our parents and we grow older.[3]

A question from a rabbi to the Responsa Committee of the Central Conference of American Rabbis, in 1980, shows how the seemingly straightforward obligation to honor a parent can be experienced as a heart-wrenching dilemma:

> If an aged parent who now lives with his family is feeble to such an extent that he would be much better cared for in a nursing home, but if he strenuously objects to leaving the

family home, what in the light of Jewish tradition can be done under these circumstances?[4]

This question—is nursing home placement of a parent, forced placement, compatible with the commandment to honor one's parents?—was raised during a time of public outrage at widely publicized scandals involving patterns of abuse, as well as government investigations into nursing home operations. In 1977 Congress had adopted Medicare and Medicaid Antifraud and Abuse Amendments. Bruce C. Vladeck's widely read book *Unloving Care* appeared in 1980.

Rabbi Solomon Freehof's response to the question is based on a passage in the Babylonian Talmud:

> It may happen that a son will feed his father the finest of food, and yet the son deserves the punishment of hell. On the other hand, it may be that the son will bind his father to the millstone to grind grain, and yet that son will deserve the blessing of Paradise. How can this be? In the first case, the father asks the son, "Where did you get all these dainties, my son?" and the son answers gruffly, "Eat and be silent like a dog eats." In the other case, the heathen king had summoned all owners of grist mills to be captured into permanent slavery, and the son says to the father (who still owns the mill), "Father, I will say that I am the owner and will go and be enslaved in your place, while you will pretend to be a mere employee who is hired to grind the grain." This son who forces his father to a miserable task in order to save him from a worse misery deserves Paradise.
>
> BT *Kiddushin* 31a

More than a thousand years after this talmudic passage was set down, the *Shulchan Aruch* (The Code of Jewish Law) offered clarification and advice:

> If the son makes the father grind at the millstone, but his intention is for the benefit of the father, to save him from a worse situation, then the son should speak words of kindness

to the heart of the father and show the father that his inten-
tion is for the father's benefit, until the father finally consents
to grind at the millstone. This son will inherit Paradise.[5]

Our first responsibility, then, is to examine our motives. Writes Rabbi
Freehof: ". . . children [who seek nursing home placement over the parent's objection] must be sure of their motives. If they are sure that their
motives are not selfish, but for the good of the parent, then it is their duty
to reason with him until he consents, if only reluctantly." He concludes
that "gentle persuasion" is the appropriate response to the parent's stren-
uous objection.[6]

Maimonides and the *Shulchan Aruch* cite a similar situation in support
of hiring others to care for a parent:

> One whose father or mother has become mentally impaired
> should try to treat them according to their mental ability with
> pity for them. But if he cannot stand it, because they have
> become too deranged, he should leave them and go, directing
> others to treat them appropriately.[7]

In the case of mental derangement, the child must arrange for others
to care for the parent; abandonment of the parent is not an option. By
analogy, according to Rabbi Langer, Jewish law permits nursing home
placement—whether or not "gentle persuasion" works—because the
negative effects of trying to care for the parent would diminish the child's
ability to show honor and reverence.[8]

> *Farewell house, and farewell home.*
> Richard Crashaw

> *You have put friend and neighbor far from me*
> *and my companions out of my sight.*
> Psalm 88:19

When new patients come in here, they often feel abandoned
by their families. They don't understand why they have to be
here. They either lash out or they become depressed. We

watch them closely. You have to move quickly, to get to know them and so that they will trust you. At the first sign from them, you must be there to respond, to get them to interact. Otherwise it's all over. You can never reach them. They will just be here and waste away.[9]

Entry into a nursing home is what sociologists call a "status passage"—a movement "from one of life's resting places to another."[10] Chief among the obstacles to accomplishing this difficult change of status is the fact that frequently "gentle persuasion" does not work, and nursing home placement is experienced as a forced move—involuntary and illegitimate. "I fall many times at home," said one distraught woman—a widow with a fraying support system—upon admission to a nursing facility. "I begged my daughter not to call the ambulance. I was not hurt [by the fall]. I was so mad when I heard the ambulance come."[11]

There can be comfort, even healing, in the act of locating one's own predicament in a larger context and, in so doing, seeing one's own life story as part of a larger narrative. The Jewish people's historical experience provides such a context for those who would bring a spiritual dimension to the issues of nursing home placement.

The prophet Jeremiah wrote in the sixth century B.C.E.:

> Alas! Lonely sits the city once great with people! She that was great among nations is become like a widow; the princess among states is become a thrall. Bitterly she weeps in the night, her cheek wet with tears. . . . Judah has gone into exile because of misery and harsh oppression. . . .
>
> Lamentations 1:1–2

The Babylonian siege of Jerusalem came to its dramatic end in 586 B.C.E. with the burning of the Holy City, the razing of Solomon's Temple, and the exile of the survivors. "By the rivers of Babylon, there we sat, sat and wept, as we thought of Zion": Psalm 137 documents the trauma of Jewish dislocation in 586 B.C.E.—our people's involuntary, illegitimate passage from homeland to "alien soil." In addition, Psalm 137 captures quintessential themes of the Jewish experience both in sixth-century B.C.E. Babylonia and in later times: suffering and hope, exile and faith, persecution and endurance.

The essential link between the personal experience of nursing home placement and the national experience of the Babylonian exile is *loss of home*. In the first instance, it takes the form of "breaking up" a house; in the second, the breakdown and ruin of God's House. These are profound losses, and they share a crucial characteristic: both are the work of uncontrollable forces—whether the enemies are external (the Babylonian army) or internal (a broken hip, dementia, diabetes, a stroke). The nursing home experience—a loss caused by "enemies"—is, indeed, the stuff that biblical laments are made of: protest, rage, depression, a feeling of abandonment, and with it all, a sense of disorientation.[12]

So keen a crisis is the loss of one's home that mortality rates among the elderly increase dramatically during the months before and after a forced move to an unfamiliar setting—especially a nursing home. Called "transfer trauma" or "relocation trauma," the problem is stress and anxiety brought on by disorientation, fear of the unknown, a sense of unpredictability, and a loss of control.

A research study at the University of Michigan in the 1970s focused on precisely this kind of stress. The researchers designed a program of orientation to new surroundings for older adults undergoing an involuntary move. The group that received the full orientation had a survival rate of 73 percent. The group that was given a more limited orientation had a survival rate of 48 percent. The message was unmistakable: potentially fatal stress can be significantly diminished by addressing the root causes of relocation trauma.[13]

The Jewish people's collective response to "relocation trauma" in biblical times can provide a spiritual model today for individuals who suffer from the disorientation caused by a forced move. Two distinct elements of that collective response emerge as a survival strategy for us. First is *verbal expression*: the articulation of grief, despair, and anger—powerfully expressed in Psalm 137. The following illustrates the point:

> At a recent conference I attended at Memorial Sloan Kettering on "Cancer and Religion," one of the presenters discussed the findings of a doctoral study in which the subjects were instructed to keep their feet in a bucket of ice, which could become very painful. The study discovered that the subject could keep his or her foot in the ice twice as long if there

was someone else in the room with whom the subject could speak and to whom the subject could complain. The study concluded that having a listening ear available made the pain more endurable.[14]

The second element is *resilience*: the people's ability to reorient itself to a new set of circumstances and realities.[15] The singer of Psalm 137 framed what is arguably the most important question in all of biblical history: "How can we sing a song of *Adonai* on alien soil?" (Psalm 137:4). The question rises from the darkness of depression and disorientation, but not hopelessness; the question contains within itself its own answer— the possibility of a new orientation: we *can* sing God's song here; we can worship God where we are. And the new orientation works because it embraces the past even as it moves in a new direction: we can pray in the Diaspora, but we face Jerusalem; we face up to the ruins. While Jerusalem remains the spiritual center, defiance and hope enable Jews to transform theology and worship after the Destruction. By the rivers of Babylon they created prayers and psalms and synagogue: a vibrant, dynamic spiritual life *outside* the Land of Israel.

At the core of our people's religious quandary—"How can we sing a song of *Adonai* on alien soil?"—is the universal question we face as individuals: how can we affirm our life stories and our values when unwanted change has disrupted our lives? If those who managed the transformation of the Jewish people in the Babylonian exile could give us advice today, they would have two lessons for us: (1) identify those things that gave your life meaning in the past; (2) plant yourself firmly in the present, while sustaining an authentic connection to the past.

The solution, then, to Psalm 137's pivotal question is *continuity between past and present.* The challenge for new nursing home residents and families—indeed, the challenge all human beings face when crisis interrupts the normal flow of life—is to identify ways to reaffirm values, engage in meaningful activities, and sustain relationships.

The religious practices of Judaism can be particularly meaningful for older adults in a nursing home. Jewish worship, study, and ritual offer opportunities to develop warm, intimate relationships with other people. Traditional religious activities create settings in which the participants can play socially significant roles (for example, synagogue honors such as an *aliyah* or opening the ark), learn new ideas and skills, and express their sense of relationship with God or share with others their struggle with God. Religious settings offer the opportunity to think and talk about things that matter. The result of all this can be a renewed sense of purpose.[16]

Furthermore, religious practice can be good for the body as well as the soul. According to the *International Journal of Psychiatry in Medicine*, ". . . people who attend weekly services have healthier immune systems than those who don't. . . . " The research involved people with Alzheimer's, depression, AIDS, and other diseases.[17]

There are many nursing homes where barely a handful of Jews reside. We may be unsure how to bring the Jewish spiritual dimension to a nursing home resident when the facility itself offers scant resources or is remote from an organized Jewish community. Congregations that are far from large cities or in places where Jewish resources are scarce provide one answer to this problem: motivated people become abundantly self-sufficient. What can you do for a Jew in a nursing home in a small town in Maine, Wyoming, or New Mexico? Or, for that matter, in some of the equally isolated facilities in Baltimore, Boston, and Los Angeles? Bring a home-baked challah and grape juice or wine; say the *Motzi* and *Kiddush*; play CDs or tapes of Israeli or klezmer music; read a Jewish story together and discuss it; decorate the room with Jewish art and objects; bring a *tzedakah* box to the room so the resident can feel like "a contributing member of society"; and bring children as often as possible. In other words, create a Jewish home! To paraphrase *Pirkei Avot*: In a place where there are no Jews, be a Jew!

When nursing home placement threatens to erect emotional walls between parent and child, we need assurance that God's blessings can still be ours. Affixing a mezuzah to the doorway of a nursing home room can be a powerful expression of that need; it is a symbol of faith and tradition—a constant reminder of the source of goodness in our lives. In a prayer for entering a nursing home, Rabbi Cary Kozberg gives us inspiration for that moment: "Amid uncertainty, may I turn to You in hope and trust."[18]

When Our Parents
Can No Longer Decide

RABBI SANDRA ROSENTHAL BERLINER

The call came at 6:00 in the morning. My mother was in the hospital. She was in excruciating pain. My father was home alone, wheelchair-bound. What were we to do? What would happen if Mom also would not be able to walk again? Would they need nursing aids? Companions? Residential care? And who would make those decisions? Mom? Dad? My sister? My brother? Myself?

Those few months during the summer were difficult and extremely challenging. Dealing with unhelpful doctors, witnessing the pain of my strong, active mother, worrying about my father, and concerns over finances kept my sister and me extremely exhausted.

My work over the past dozen years or so as a hospice chaplain, and as a chaplain to older adults, did not completely prepare me for the whirl-wind of decisions that my family needed to face in light of this latest catastrophe. And catastrophe it was! It took several long weeks before a definite diagnosis was made. My mother was given all kinds of medications, which caused her confusion and barely eased her pain.

And, at the same time, my father was home alone, attempting to cope without his wife, who had been *his* primary caregiver for the past several years.

We were fortunate. My mother is walking again, nearly pain-free (thank God!), and my father is using a walker. Both of them live inde-pendently in their own apartment with the help of a daily companion who cleans, does laundry, and drives. For now, calm is restored. Yet, this experience left all of us feeling vulnerable to whatever might happen next to my parents down the road.

I know that my family and I are not the only ones who are surprised at the magnitude of being responsible for aging parents. So many of us take for granted the health and well-being of our parents. As young children, we look toward our parents as our life-givers and caretakers. Mom and Dad are the ones who teach us to walk, to talk, to swim, and to play ball. They transmit their sacred religious values, their morals, and their ethics. Our parents are the ones who take care of us when we're sick, who dry our tears when we're hurt, and who cheer us on when we succeed. When we are young, our parents seem powerful, strong, and nearly immortal.

Yet, the reality for most of us is that, our parents *will* grow old. We pray that they will be able to *schlep* the *naches* of grandchildren, enjoy retirement, and know the satisfaction of a life well lived. However, the process of growing older can sometimes be different from those bright expectations. There may come a time when our parents need us to step in as caregivers and decision makers for *them*.

Decision making for parents is generally an emotion-laden, difficult task. Roles become reversed, with the children becoming the caregivers and the people in charge. When there is more than one child involved, sibling issues arise. Sometimes financial issues loom. The way in which we approach the awesome task of deciding whether to place a parent in a nursing home, to remove a parent from a respirator, to continue dialysis, or to stop aggressive cancer treatment needs to be based on a combination of Jewish teachings, the best medical advice available, knowledge of what parents desire, and ultimately love.

> *Honor thy father and thy mother, that thy days may be long upon the land which* Adonai *thy God giveth thee.*
>
> Exodus 20:12

The Torah tells us that we should honor our parents, yet it does not state specific ways in which we should follow that precept. The Talmud, however, does provide some help. From Tractate *Kiddushin* we learn: "Of what does honor for parents consist? In providing for them food and drink, in clothing them, in giving them shoes for their feet, in helping them to enter or leave the house" (BT *Kiddushin* 31b–32a).

In Jewish life, we are taught to honor our parents, obey them, and be humble before them. Notice that nowhere in Jewish law is there the command "to love" one's parents. Even the Rabbis knew that while one could not legislate feelings, Jews had an inherent responsibility toward their parents. This view is consonant with the idea of Judaism as a religion of mitzvot, sacred commandments. In most of Judaism, what we *do* is paramount to what we *feel*. And while love is often a motivating force toward fulfilling one's filial obligations, if it is absent, as Jews we are still commanded to make sure that our parents are treated with the honor and respect due them.

Ideally, every individual should possess a living will and a durable power of attorney. These documents express the wishes of our loved ones even when they no longer can speak for themselves. The living will states clearly the preferences for such situations as heroic measures, life support, and medical treatment. The durable power of attorney gives children (or whoever is the designated decision maker) the ability to proceed on their parents' behalf. Both documents are extremely helpful in any decision making. If we know that Mom would not want to remain on a ventilator, kept alive though technically brain-dead, then the decision to "not resuscitate" is clear.

Throughout the Jewish world, there are many models of preparing these types of advanced directives.[1] However, many people do not have living wills or even durable powers of attorney. As they suffer with dementia and confusion, or if they slip into a coma or noncommunicative state, health-care decisions often need to be made by children.

One of the most difficult and painful decisions for an adult child is placing a parent in a nursing home. Though there are now many excellent senior care facilities, from personal care, to assisted living, to skilled care, it is still wrenching to have one's mother or father move from his or her home to a one-room or half-room existence.

When a parent is placed in a nursing home, taken from familiar surroundings, having to give up precious possessions and belongings, as well as independence, it can be a devastating loss. One woman once said to me, "It broke my heart to give up all my books!" Another said, "They're always telling me what to do!" And still others have commented to me about the lack of privacy, about missing certain foods, and neighbors.

Though the Talmud commands us to provide shelter for our parents, it does not mean necessarily in our own homes. In the *Kitzur Shulchan Aruch*, there is a section that advises, "If one's father or mother becomes demented, the son would endeavor to act with them in accordance with their mental condition, until God will have mercy on them. However, if the son can no longer bear it because of their aggravated condition, he may leave them and delegate others to take care of them."[2]

Many loving children have placed their parents in nursing homes, visited regularly, insisted on excellent care, *and* felt guilty throughout. But, as the *Kitzur Shulchan Aruch* continues in the next paragraph, "A man is forbidden to place a burdensome yoke upon his children. . . ."[3] Therefore, families who do end up placing their parents in long-term residential centers might find comfort from knowing that in so doing they are fulfilling their Jewish obligations, as well as doing what may very well be in the best interests of their parents. Since we honor our parents by providing for their needs, sometimes long-term residential care is the only option. A patient suffering from Alzheimer's who wanders from his house in the middle of the night needs round-the-clock care, which his children cannot provide.

I remember working with a family as a hospice chaplain when such an occasion arose. Sam was a ninety-year-old man. He had lived independently most of his life. After his second wife passed away, he slowly deteriorated, both physically and mentally. He became confused, and would not eat or take his medications. His two sons were responsible for his care, and both had families of their own. Although they visited frequently, they feared for the time when Dad would have an accident or a stroke and they would not know it. Therefore, they decided to place him in a Jewish long-term care facility. Throughout the time that Sam lived there, his family visited, brought gifts, and took him out when they could. They attended religious services with him, as well. Sam's sons did the best they could for him given the circumstances of his health and mental status.

Though Sam's sons had moments of guilt, they were generally able to derive comfort from knowing that they were observing the mitzvah of *kibud av va-eim* "honoring one's father and mother." They showed reverence for their father by ensuring him safe and dignified care when they were unable to provide it. The decision was not an easy one, yet assessing the alternatives, the children made the best choice they could for their father at that time.

The removal of life support is another difficult issue caregivers may confront. Sometimes, parents become gravely ill from a stroke, heart attack, or some other disabling affliction that renders them incapable of communicating. In such times, it becomes the awesome responsibility of children to make decisions about when to terminate treatment. In Judaism, each person is regarded as having been created *b'tzelem ud'mut Elohim,*" "in the image and likeness of God" (Genesis 1:26–27). We each possess the divine spark inherent in every human being. As inevitable as it is that we will all one day die, it is not up to us to personally decide when to end life.

When faced with the decision of removing life support, whether it be a ventilator, kidney dialysis, or other means of sustaining life, adult children need to consider the Jewish views concerning those acts, as well as the ethics of caring for parents discussed above. Dr. Benjamin Freedman writes, "The verse prohibiting striking a parent, prohibits causing pain; in general, Jewish tradition treats psychological pain—anguish—at least as seriously as it does physical pain".[4] The Torah also teaches, "He who insults his father or his mother shall be put to death" (Exodus 21:17). The Hebrew word for "insult" is *kalal,* or "to make light of." Dr. Freedman asserts that this means to treat someone lightly, without dignity. Thus, when making decisions concerning the treatment of parents, we are urged to follow that commandment and not to let our parents suffer.[5]

Judaism absolutely forbids suicide, physician-assisted suicide, and euthanasia. Yet, deciding to let our parents be in the hands of God, in a dignified, pain-free manner, serves the higher order of *kibud av va-eim,* "honoring one's father and one's mother." As a hospice rabbi, I have faced many such momentous decisions with families. The decision to discontinue life support is made with extreme difficulty and wrenching pain.

I'll never forget being in the hospital with Harold and his family. Harold was a 75-year-old man. He had survived heart attacks, bypass surgery, and other assorted illnesses. For the last year of his life, he was in and out of the hospital frequently. His sons and wife were constantly by his side. The last time Harold was in the hospital, he fell into a coma. He was nonresponsive, yet the ventilator continued to keep him breathing. Without a living will, his family was uncertain of his wishes. When the doctor told them that Harold's chances of coming out of the coma were extremely minimal, he offered the option of shutting down the ventilator.

Together, his children, his wife, and I discussed the aspects of what life meant to Harold. One of the most difficult issues for the sons was feeling like they would be "killing" their father; a common feeling for children in this situation. As the chaplain and as a rabbi, it was important for me to understand Harold's and his family's philosophy of what made life meaningful and to offer the Jewish "voice."

There was controversy between the two brothers. One felt uncomfortable about shutting off the ventilator, as he did not want to "play God." The other son thought that his father would not have wanted to "live" that way, as Harold had been such a vital, active participant throughout his life. Since there was no hope of recovery or even regaining consciousness, the family ultimately based their decision on the Jewish values of honoring one's parents and preserving their dignity. There was nothing invasive about stopping the ventilator. When it was shut off, I asked the family to gather together for prayers and comfort. We offered the *Vidui* (the final confession), and Harold died two days later.

Harold's family had been actively involved in their synagogue for many years. They were firmly grounded in their Jewish culture and faith. There was adequate justification for choosing either way in this case, yet ultimately, the decision to provide for their father's dignity in the face of death prevailed. Having based their decision on Jewish values, with the support of a Jewish chaplain, brought comfort and closure to their painful situation.

Another difficult issue that confronts caregivers is end of life care. At the end of life, when a parent has a terminal illness such as cancer, congestive heart failure, or anterior lateral sclerosis (Lou Gehrig's disease), there are other issues to consider. Factors such as pain control, spiritual comfort, and emotional and physical support all need to be addressed. The decisions here are not all that different from the scenarios mentioned above. The parent's mental competency, physical abilities, finances, and proximity of children to the parent all need to be taken into consideration.

One option might be skilled care placement, as has been previously discussed. Another might be hospitalization as needed. Another possibility could be for the parent to move in with the adult child. No matter what interim solution is reached, the highly charged issues of death and dying are always present. Eventually decisions will need to be made in these situations that specifically relate not to living with or managing the disease, but to death.

One method of dealing with people dealing with terminal illness is hospice care. Hospice is a concept that has become quite popular in the United States over the past twenty years. It is a philosophy of care that provides for pain relief and emotional and spiritual support to enable patients to live out the remainder of their lives as meaningfully as possible to the very end. The idea of hospice care is not to hasten death, nor to prolong suffering. Hospice provides comfort for both the patient and families until the very end, often in the patient's own home. This provides for the opportunity to care for parents while still receiving help and support from the hospice team.

Hospice care fits beautifully within the framework of the Jewish approach to the end of life. In the *Shulchan Aruch*, we read that while it is forbidden to hasten death, still we are permitted to remove an external cause "that prevents the departure of the soul, such as the noise of some pounding, that cause may be removed, since this is not a direct deed to hasten the end."[6] Through the use of hospice care, the family and patient do not prevent death, yet offer comfort measures through pain medication, relaxation techniques, counseling, and prayer.

The decision to opt for hospice can be difficult. It can feel like simply giving up. However, when there is nothing else that can be done medically, hospice can play a very significant role at the end of life. Having been a hospice rabbi for thirteen years, I have been involved with many patients and families at this time of their lives. When is aggressive medical treatment "enough"? At what point do we allow our parents the time to live their lives as pain-free as possible and as dignified as possible?

Usually, a physician will suggest hospice when all avenues to cure have been tried. One family I worked with agreed to place their father on hospice care after he had suffered a long bout of chemotherapy and several operations. When the children were assured that the concept of hospice care was in consonance with Jewish tradition and that their father would be gently cared for, hospice seemed perfect. With hospice, their father would be able to remain in his own home, in his familiar and familial surroundings. His pain would be controlled, and with the involvement and proximity of people who loved and cared for him, he could make some sort of meaning out of every day he had left. In this case, the children provided for the care and sustenance of their father, as well as the honor and dignity commanded by the Torah.

There are countless other examples of situations where adult children might find themselves in the role of caregiver for parents who can no longer make their own decisions. As parents age and their needs for help increase, Jewish tradition demands that children take a positive and critical role in caregiving. The commandment of honoring parents means so much more than lip service of respect. The decisions that must be made regarding the care of aging parents are difficult and often even wrenching. But if we make our decisions based on the commandments and teachings provided by Jewish tradition, we can find some comfort in knowing that we have provided ways for our parents to live out their lives with meaning and dignity, with love and respect.

A Granddaughter's Story:
One Family's Decision-Making Process

⚜

Dr. Adina Kalet

"Please call Dr. Kamner, you know him from medical school, he needs consent to do a colonoscopy on Grandma. . . ." My father's voice on the phone that summer day was uncharacteristically tense and sad. I knew immediately that this was more than the routine request of his "daughter the doctor." It was rare for him to ask me to intervene with another physician this directly; usually he would just inform me about some new medical development or ask about getting a second opinion. This time he was not just calling to let me know he met someone who knew me. He was asking me to step up to the plate, both as a physician and a granddaughter.

I am not the *only* doctor in my family. My uncle has a Ph.D. in electrical engineering—as he reminds me from time to time with a twinkle in his eye—but I am *the* physician among a family of smart, educated people. This is a complex role, one they should prepare you for in medical school but don't. I have learned through experience that the most effective approach to caring for family members is to resist the desire to be the doctor and focus instead on ensuring they have a good relationship with a trustworthy, thorough physician. I make the match and try to stay informed but out of the way. Then there are the other times when the stakes are high, the health care is fragmented, and the medical situation is complex and emotionally challenging. The last few weeks of my grandmother's life was such a time.

Grandma, Sara Rabey Kalet, the indisputable matriarch of our small family, was a Jewish woman whose life was shaped and defined by the events of the time in which she lived. Born in Poland at the turn of the century, she immigrated to New York City just before World War II. The siblings she had every hope of bringing over as soon as possible were torn from her by the Holocaust. This tragedy defined but did not destroy her adult life. "Little Grandma," as we called her because of her diminutive five-foot frame, was the quintessential Balabusta. She cooked and cleaned and sewed with great skill and intensity. She and Grandpa lived modestly in the south Bronx, raised their two sons, and lived to see their five grandchildren into adulthood. Eventually she became frail and lost some of her vigor. Grandpa died when she was in her seventies, and living alone became increasingly difficult. One day, while home alone, she tripped over a rug and broke her hip. She lay on the floor banging with a stick for hours until someone heard and broke into the apartment. The convalescence that followed the hip replacement surgery proved painful and difficult, sapping her of her courage. Eventually she asked to be in a nursing home. She did not want to be alone or to "burden" her children.

By the time of my father's call she had lived in the Jewish Home for the Aged for many years. She had long since lost decisional capacity—the ability to understand and participate in a complex choice about her own medical care. She had been a no-nonsense, practical woman. Now she was anxious, confused, and mute when faced with simple choices. It had been years since she had handed over the managing of her affairs to her sons and daughters-in-law. Now she could no longer participate in important choices that required her to understand the nature of procedures and to weigh risks against benefits. Legally, it was my father's role, as her designated health-care proxy, to make all her decisions.

After a short conversation with the gastroenterologist, I found out that Grandma had been "dwindling" over the past few weeks. She had stopped eating, was losing weight, and had blood in her stool, although she otherwise seemed comfortable. On hearing this story, a common, familiar, and worrisome one to any experienced internist, I swooned, teetering on the dividing wall between granddaughter and doctor. But I recovered my balance enough to participate in the usual doctor-doctor talk.

"I don't practice in a nursing home. Tell me, what would it take to perform the colonoscopy?" I managed to ask.

He answered perfunctorily in the monotone he probably used whenever explaining something this routine. Meanwhile I imagined the pain and disorientation such a trip to the hospital would likely cause someone in my grandma's condition.

"Given that she is so frail and has recently become bedridden, it would require an ambulance 'transfer' to the hospital [read: strapped to a gurney for hours] for the 'prep' [read: an all-fluid diet that 'cleaned out the colon' by causing watery diarrhea], the procedure with mild sedation if she couldn't cooperate [which she couldn't], and then a 'transfer' back. . . ."

"What do you think is most likely?" I asked, knowing the answer but not wanting to be the first to say it.

"Well, I am almost certain this is colon cancer . . . it's possible there's some bowel ischemia, but then she would be more uncomfortable, then again the blood could be a red herring and there could be neoplasm [read: cancer] somewhere else. . . ." He spoke to me like any doctor might about any patient. In doctor parlance, this is paradoxically the ultimate sign of respect and caring for a physician family member, since he was speaking in the familiar form of doctor-dialect, being careful not to talk down to me or to soften his language in any way.

Then I expressed a feeling we both found challenging to consider. "So why pursue this? She is very frail but comfortable, there is no evidence she is in pain, the colonoscopy could be challenging and uncomfortable, surgery would be very risky, and she's likely to die from whatever this is soon . . . she is ninety-two years old and with a profound Alzheimer's dementia. . . ."

"Better to know isn't it. . . ?" He inserted before I could play out the entire scenario, expressing the intolerance of uncertainty that makes our profession what it is, both for the good and for the bad.

I began to envision what was in store for my grandmother and, more important in some ways, for my father and uncle. Suddenly, I was hell-bent on slowing our momentum down this "slippery slope" long enough to have the discussion with my family. I asked him to hold off a few more days. I promised to get back to him. He protested a little, but agreed to wait.

Was it best to know? I was doubtful. As a physician I was all too familiar with what was likely to happen to her, a frail, very confused old woman in an acute care hospital, if we simply let the physicians pursue a diagnosis. As her granddaughter, I wanted my grandmother to have a pain-free and dignified end of her life. In my experience with my own patients,

I knew that Jewish families generally want to know all that there is to know, valuing and drawing comfort from the information, willing to suffer some discomfort in the pursuit of the truth. Certainly in my family, while no one would want Grandma to undergo unnecessary suffering, we are not afraid to face the truth. But was this right?

My desire was to protect Grandma's dignity and to respect my father and uncle's wishes. I realized that I had been grieving the loss of my "Little Grandma" for a long time. It had been two years since she had recognized me or asked about my life, more than that since she had shared a recipe or a sewing tip. But despite the fact that she had been fading away, she was still at the center of both of her son's daily lives. Their devotion to her was steadfast and uncomplicated. I didn't want them left with doubts or guilt or horrible images of their mother's death.

I consulted with my most trusted colleague, my husband Mark, who is also a physician. He helped me make and carry out a plan. I had spent enough time on the phone discussing this with my father, uncle, brother, and cousins to know that everyone had his or her own unique perspective, and it became clear that we needed to have the discussion as a group. Whether we liked it or not, we had many difficult choices to make in the days to come. I wanted to make sure everyone understood the issues and that we agreed on the goals of care. While the decision was my father's and my uncle's to make, it was assumed they were not going to do so in isolation. We called a family meeting.J180

There was no precedent in my family for formal and serious "meetings." Even on serious occasions we are informal, love to banter and tell jokes and stories (again and again), avoid the personally challenging, argue the politically challenging, and never sit together without food. So Mark and I drew on our professional experience with conducting such meetings for our patients and their families. We agreed that he should run the meeting so that I was free to be a family member. The next evening in our dinning room, over coffee and cake, Mark laid it all out as gently and calmly as possible to my father, uncle, and aunt. My brother and his wife could not be there, but gave us their blessings. My cousins were all in Israel but would be informed and consulted by phone and e-mail.

"She is ninety-three years old, her mind is mostly gone, and given the clinical situation—the weight loss, blood in stool, and loss of appetite—it is likely she has a very serious diagnosis, very likely colon cancer." Our family had never been so still and quiet as when Mark spoke.

"The choice at this point is whether to know or not know. The treatment for this cancer is surgery. We would need to figure out whether she would have chosen surgery—given the risks of anesthesia and hospitalization," he said, to establish that the goal was to determine what she would most likely have chosen for herself if she could choose.

"She is still a person, we can't just . . . ," my uncle said in a quieter voice than I have ever heard come from him. The realization had hit him that Mark was saying that there was no good choice, only a best one.

Mark continued to lay it out, using probabilities and technical explanations when he was asked to, trying not to overwhelm anyone. We talked about what a colonoscopy would mean. We answered uncomfortable questions about what it would be like to die of cancer and what was likely to be the hospital course. We talked about what the nursing home would and would not do for Grandma. We talked about what we each believed Grandma could understand at this point, and we all agreed that we did not believe she could understand much at all, but if she could, she would have refused any further tests and would have asked to be allowed to die peacefully.

From time to time someone would turn to me and ask, "What do you think?" Although I was pretty clear by then that I felt we should stop all diagnostic testing and provide aggressive palliative care in familiar surroundings, I felt unable to admit this out loud. I was feeling very much like the little girl I had always been in this circle, precocious and articulate but not responsible for anything serious. At the same time, I was concerned that my opinion as a physician would carry too much weight. I wanted us to do what Grandma would have wanted if she could have said, and what her sons could live with. I also was reluctant to take responsibility for pressuring them to do something with which they could not reconcile. So I was uncharacteristically inarticulate and unopinionated.

By the end, it was clear to everyone present that while less intervention could be the "right" choice, "not doing" everything possible to take care of their mother was an almost unbearable thought for the brothers. We were stuck and needed more time.

When I called the primary doctor at the nursing home the next day, he informed me that he had ordered an abdominal CAT scan of Grandma, which revealed a large "intraluminal obstructing lesion consistent with colon cancer in the sigmoid colon." I asked him why he went ahead and ordered a test that required a trip to the hospital and an hour on a very hard table in a cold room.

"Because it was a way to proceed without having to obtain

consent from the family," he replied, since consent for a CAT scan was covered under the general consent for treatment given when my grandmother entered the home. I was furious but not surprised by his avoidance of discussion with the family. I knew it was his responsibility to do this for us, that it is the right thing to do, and that he wasn't going to do it. Some physicians avoid this kind of interaction with patients and families for a variety of different reasons. At the same time, I couldn't help but be relieved that the facts had been clarified— there was a large tumor in Grandma's colon. He also informed me that she would be admitted to the hospital for a biopsy to confirm the diagnosis. Since we were not yet clear as a family on how we wanted to proceed, she went to the hospital.

After a series of delays and bumbles, after my Grandma had spent a week in the hospital without a diagnosis, the surgeon asked for consent for a feeding tube. This was the moment I faced my anger at and disappointment with my profession for allowing so predictable a hospital course for this "nursing home transfer" and for not taking on the difficult discussions with the family. As the daughter, I was sad for my father and uncle, who clearly didn't want their mother to die, and I had been struggling with how active and forceful to be with my family and my grandmother's physicians. Luckily my professional training had prepared me to think through and act in the face of these sort of dilemmas. I was finally ready to sit everyone down in the waiting room of the hospital and make a clear statement.

"She is dying. We need to decide how we want her to die." By now everyone had had enough experience to make a choice. We had her returned to the nursing home, where she quickly became less agitated and more comfortable in the familiar surroundings.

Wanting to make sure that our wishes would be followed, I tracked down the nursing home physician and told him, "We want aggressive comfort care—adequate pain meds, no unnecessary tests." He took an audible deep breath, made no empathic or understanding comments, and briskly referred me to his boss, the medical director of the home, to convene an ethics committee meeting, which was necessary before he "felt comfortable" following our wishes.

Again my professional experience came into play. I knew that in order to be effective, we needed to present clear and convincing evidence that what we were asking for was what Grandma would have wanted. So on the morning of the meeting, two days before Yom Kippur, we sat together over breakfast and composed our family statement.

During the meeting of the ethics committee, I sat among twelve people, the nurses and doctors involved in her care, a rabbi, a social worker, the medical director, my father, and my uncle. Information was presented in a very stark, matter-of-fact way. We had decided I would speak formally for the family. It was important to me to be articulate in my presentation of why following our wishes was both medically appropriate and the morally and ethically right way to proceed, because I wanted my father and uncle to feel they were doing right by their mother and I wanted to be both granddaughter and physician to my beloved grandmother. It was my turn.

"My grandmother has lived a long life. Toward the end, she frequently talked of dying, she felt she had suffered enough pain and that she could now let go." I took a deep breath to hold back the tears. "She survived very many tragic losses, including the death of her father, which left her to lead the family business and run the family, then immigration to a new country, leaving behind her siblings and mother. The most dramatic was the horrible discovery that they had all perished at the hand of Hitler. Finally, the loss of her husband of fifty years, a fractured hip, and a long and painful last fifteen years during which time she . . . she had many joyful times and a family who love her very much, saw her grandchildren grow to adulthood; she was able to be at my wedding, she held her first great-grandchild. But in the last few years she has gradually lost touch with her memories, she no longer recognizes her grandchildren, she often seems as if she is terrified and lost . . . all she is able to say is 'Help, help, help. . . .' I looked around the room. The nursing staff were nodding their heads; they knew what I was saying was true.

"At this time we believe that if she could decide for herself, she would no longer choose to go on. We believe she would have refused any further curative care, especially given that cure is very unlikely and the treatments are harsh. So what we do want is for her to receive aggressive comfort care focused on anticipating, avoiding, and relieving pain and suffering."

There was a little discussion among the group but no debate. Each member was invited to speak; few did. Finally the medical director ended by assuring us that Grandma would be cared for in the way we asked. We walked out quietly together and went to her bedside.

Grandma did well for a couple of weeks. At first she ate small amounts of food and water and then stopped. No blood was drawn or tests done, and she died peacefully, in her sleep.

Shivah was a satisfying time; I could be the granddaughter again. There were friends and family, photographs and stories, tears and laughter. Family dynamics returned to the usual. I was no longer needed as the expert or interpreter, no longer the spokesperson. I was satisfied knowing that I helped ensure Grandma a "good death." I was glad to know that we followed what we were sure she would have wanted and that my father and uncle felt they had done the right thing.

꩜

On Suffering

RABBI ALAN HENKIN

> Dear God, I care not why I suffer. I wish only to know that
> I suffer for Your sake.
> —*Rabbi Levi Yitzchak of Berditchev*

Suffering is both the most universal of human experiences and the most personal. Throughout our people's long history, we Jews have wrestled with suffering, its ubiquity and its meaning. As long ago as the Creation story in Genesis 1–3, we have sought to answer such impenetrable questions as, Why is there death? Why must women give birth in pain? Why must men toil so hard to survive?

The conundrum of suffering for all religious people is this: if God is all-powerful, morally good, and concerned with human welfare, why does God allow, or even cause, people to suffer so terribly? This paradox, called theodicy, constitutes the major problematic question of all faiths. Why did God allow tens of thousands of innocent people to die in earthquakes in Turkey? Why did God allow tens of thousands to die in floods in Venezuela? Why did God allow millions of people to die in Nazi death camps? Why did God allow my mother to get Alzheimer's disease? Why does God allow me to hurt so much from my fibromyalgia?

We Jews have earned Ph.D.'s in suffering. Starvation, famine, disease, epidemic, exile, torture, war, terrorism, genocide, and more have all been visited upon us. In sacred Scripture as well as *New York Times* best-sellers, we have articulated our responses to such pain. In a sense, our entire medieval mystical movement, the Kabbalah, is an effort to explicate the suffering created by the exile from Spain in 1492. Our Jewish bona fides on suffering are impeccable.

For many the moral, religious, and philosophical issues raised by suffering are remote and abstract. Yet when we witness seemingly pointless and excruciating suffering in our own family, the issues become all too real. In my own family, despite our best efforts to help, we watched powerlessly as my brother descended into the hell of drug addiction, which ended only when he overdosed one May morning. My brother's pain and the pain that his untimely death caused for his widow, his three young children, our parents, and his brothers and sister continue to roil within our family, occasionally erupting in family dysfunction and outbursts of sorrow. The personal and familial ramifications of suffering can be brutal and destructive, unless we find a coherent way to deal with it.

Suffering in the Bible

The classic biblical understanding of suffering is punishment. In this view, suffering occurs because individuals or groups have sinned against God by not following the commandments. Deuteronomy 11:16–17 illustrates this: "Take care not be lured away to serve other gods and bow to them. For *Adonai*'s anger will flare up against you, and God will shut up the skies so that there will be no rain and the ground will not yield its produce; and you will soon perish from the good land that *Adonai* is assigning to you." Just as the Torah regards natural disasters such as drought and famine as punishment, so too does it regard such humanly engineered suffering as military defeat and exile as punishment. Not just communities but individuals too are punished for their sins. Miriam was stricken with a skin disease for speaking ill of her brother Moses (Numbers 12) and even Moses himself was refused entry into the Promised Land because of his disobedience of God (Numbers 20). In the latter case the punishment seems so utterly disproportionate to the offense that it has exercised Jewish commentators for millennia. Although it may be difficult for us to accept this model of suffering as punishment, it at least provides us with a coherent theological explanation: human suffering is part of God's plan, and its purpose is to exact retribution for our misdeeds.

The Jewish Bible is a compendium of many genres of holy literature. Wisdom literature makes up one such genre. We define biblical wisdom literature as that which focuses on the individual and his or her social relationships, rather than religion and ritual obligations. Among the major works of wisdom literature in the Bible are Job, Proverbs, and Ecclesiastes. These are collected in a part of our Jewish Scripture called the *K'tuvim*, or Writings. Wisdom literature presents a view of suffering that is difficult to generalize. For example, take Ecclesiastes, a somewhat radical book of wisdom known as *Kohelet* in Hebrew. The author of *Kohelet* admits time and again that no one can understand the workings of the universe.[1] Kohelet writes, "I have observed the business that God gave man to be concerned with: He brings everything to pass precisely at its time; He also puts eternity in their mind, but without man ever guessing, from first to last, all the things that God brings to pass" (Ecclesiastes 3:10–11). For Kohelet, trying to understand God's logic of reward and punishment is futile; we are better off simply accepting what life offers us, the good and the bad, without reading too much into it.

Similarly, the Book of Job offers a view of suffering that is unconventional by the Torah's standards. "The Book of Job introduces two new elements into the picture [of suffering]. First, it highlights the fate of an individual human being; second it breaks completely with the doctrine of suffering as divine retribution."[2] An utterly righteous man, Job loses his children, his possessions, and his health in quick succession, because God has handed Job over to the Satan for testing. As Job comes to grips with his suffering, he rejects as platitudes the usual explanations. Finally, in the last four chapters of the book, Job receives an "explanation" for his suffering from God. God appears to Job in a whirlwind and thunders at him, "Where were you when I laid the earth's foundations? . . . Have you ever commanded the day to break? . . . Have you penetrated to the sources of the sea, or walked in the recesses of the deep?" (Job 38:4–16). In other words, God's purposes are beyond human comprehension. Human perception fails when it bumps up against God's grandeur and majesty. "Suffering is a part of God's complex plan; it has no further explanation."[3] Both *Kohelet* and Job leave us with a frightening thought: from a human point of view, suffering is capricious.

Suffering in the Rabbinic Period

When the biblical period closed around the year 200 B.C.E., Judaism gradually moved into the rabbinic period. With the destruction of the Temple in Jerusalem in 70 C.E. and the end of its sacrificial cult, the Rabbis and their predecessors were faced with the task of reconstructing Judaism under dramatically different circumstances. New rituals, like the Passover seder, and new institutions, like the synagogue and the rabbinate itself, were adapted to ensure the survival of Judaism. New beliefs also came into being to inspire a semblance of continuity within the discontinuity caused by the upheavals of the first century.

The rabbinic understanding of suffering in some ways maintains the Torah's view of suffering as punishment, but in other ways departs from it drastically. For example, some Rabbis still understood suffering as punishment, but, going beyond the Torah, they believed that the punishment one experienced had a purpose beyond mere retribution. "Chastisements wipe out all a man's wickedness," says the Talmud in *B'rachot* 5a. "Sufferings propitiate God as much as sacrifices," wrote George Foot Moore in 1927.[4] "Beloved is suffering, for as sacrifices are atoning, so is suffering atoning," suggests a rabbinic midrash (*Sifrei* 73b). Thus one rabbinic elaboration of the Bible's notion that suffering represents punishment is that the punishment of suffering redeems the sufferer from sin.[5]

A related rabbinic twist on the meaning of suffering is that suffering is an opportunity for self-scrutiny. "When a person sees that he is being chastised, let him examine his ways," the Talmud teaches (*B'rachot* 5a). If suffering is a product of punishment, then if one suffers, one must be being punished for something; searching one's soul for sin becomes a way to eliminate both the sin and the punishment. "There is a didactic element in this explanation insofar as it encourages man to refrain from sin in order to avoid suffering," argues Steven Schwarzschild.[6] Yet another rabbinic interpretation of suffering is that of "chastisements of love." According to the Talmud (*B'rachot* 5a), God brings suffering to those whom God loves best. Suffering is not seen as punishment, but rather as an expression of God's love. God only tests those whose loyalty and devotion mean the most to God. Thus, if one suffers, one must remain steadfast in one's faith.

Rabbi and philosopher David Hartman has written extensively on the rabbinic understanding of suffering.[7] Hartman believes that the Rabbis' major innovation in handling the problem of suffering was to shift the discussion away from philosophical theology toward religious anthropology. That is, the Rabbis did not so much want to talk about God's role in evil and suffering as to talk about the Jew's response to suffering within the covenantal framework. For example, Hartman cites the martyrdom of Rabbi Akiva around 135 C.E. According to the Jerusalem Talmud (*Sotah* 5:5) when Rabbi Akiva was tortured by the Romans, he discovered an insight into the *V'ahavta*, the Torah's command to love God from Deuteronomy 6:5. "Rather than focus on repentance and on suffering in this world in order to receive reward in the next, Akiva interpreted his own suffering as an occasion to realize his great religious dream to love God unconditionally with a passion that transcended the normal human instinct of self-preservation."[8] For Hartman, then, the Rabbis tried to redirect suffering, even their own considerable suffering, into an effort to deepen their understanding of Torah and mitzvot.[9] Suffering thus becomes an opportunity for strengthening our Jewish fealty to God and the covenant.

Serious problems inhere in all these rabbinic approaches to suffering. Whether we understand suffering to be punishment for the sake of retribution or punishment for the sake of atonement, we are still left with the tragic case of the suffering of innocents. How does the suffering of an infant balance the child's sins or bring about the baby's repentance? Or again, why does God need to test with suffering those whom God loves; does not God already know the extent of their faith without resorting to such measures? Similarly we can ask of David Hartman, how does the shift from talking about suffering in terms of God to talking about suffering in terms of people really obviate the "why" questions? Just because Jews have used their trials as paths to greater insight into themselves and their God, they have not given up the problem of why they must suffer in the first place. The Holocaust like nothing else, has thoroughly undermined the adequacy of all these solutions to the problem of suffering.

Some Modern Views

Numerous modern Jewish thinkers have taken up the problem of suffering,[10] and the Holocaust has given this issue of suffering flesh-and-blood urgency. Among those who wrestle with the meaning of the Holocaust, we can find a broad range of responses. At one extreme are representatives of ultra-Orthodox Jewry, like Rabbi Schach, who invoke the classical reward-and-punishment doctrine by blaming our peoples' sufferings on their sins, especially that of assimilation, committed in Europe. At the other extreme, Richard Rubenstein claims that our facile, biblical-rabbinic conception of God has died and that the suffering endured during the Holocaust occurred because of the impersonal, natural processes of the universe and human evil.[11]

Between the extremes a tenuous consensus has emerged that affirms both human freedom and the laws of nature, on the one hand, and God's love and compassion for humanity, on the other. We cannot uphold a God who both dramatically intercedes in human affairs *and* grants true human freedom at the same time. We cannot avow both a God who miraculously intervenes in nature, and a reliable, predictable universe simultaneously. One way or another, Jewish thinkers in this middle ground assert that out of love or out of respect for human freedom or out of reasons we cannot fathom, God limits the domain of divine activity and providence. Because God restricts the divine direction of human actions and the universe, we enjoy genuine free will, which often entails the making of evil decisions, creating suffering within the human family. At the same time, the universe operates according to its own laws, which, from a human point of view, often result in devastating consequences like earthquakes or cancer.

What, then, is God's role in our lives for these theologians? In Rabbi Harold Kushner's 1981 reflection on his son's death, *When Bad Things Happen to Good People*, he expresses his belief that

> God may not prevent calamity, but He gives us the strength and the perseverance to overcome it. . . . We love Him because He is God, because He is the author of all the beauty and the order around us, the source of our strength and the hope and courage within us, and of other people's strength and hope and courage with which we are helped in our time of need.[12]

Similarly, for Rabbi Kushner prayer becomes a way to get in touch with the power of God within us.

I believe that God gives us strength and patience and hope, renewing our spiritual resources when they run dry. . . . One of the things that constantly reassures me that God is real, and not just an idea that religious leaders made up, is the fact that people who pray for strength, hope and courage so often find resources of strength, hope and courage that they did not have before.[13]

Other contemporary writers agree that although God cannot or will not curtail human evil or natural disasters, God does stand with us in our sorrow and our pain. Rabbi David Wolpe, for example, writes, "In the end, however, the Jewish position has always been to understand that, however close, there is a gap between human beings and God, and we cannot finally understand His intentions or designs. Therefore we pray."[14] Rabbi Naomi Levy echoes this notion, "But I do believe it is God who enables us to return to life after tragedy—not by eradicating all evil but by giving us the strength and the courage to face evil and to combat it. By giving us the capacity to appreciate the miracles that surround us each day, the conscience to choose good over evil, the compassion to extend our hands to those who are suffering."[15]

Our Predicament

So what does this brief survey of the various Jewish understandings of sufferings mean to us as caregivers? First of all, we learn that while we Jews have known terrible suffering through the ages and have made it a central issue in our religious and theological lives, we cannot explain it any better than anyone else. In the last analysis, suffering is a mystery; at bottom, suffering is something inexplicable and incomprehensible. Despite our very best attempts, we can never ultimately answer the "why" question. For instance, even if we fully grasped the total biochemical, genetic, and environmental processes in breast cancer, we could still ask the "why" question: why did God so structure the universe that these processes occur and cause so much misery? The wisdom writers of the Bible were right: suffering is beyond human knowledge and apprehension.

Judaism, as far back as the Torah, sees suffering as an ineradicable fact of human existence. This is the import of God's curse of Adam and Eve for their disobedience: "'I will make most severe your pangs in child-bearing; in pain you shall bear children. . . . By the sweat of your brow shall you get bread to eat, until you return to the ground'" (Genesis 3:16, 19). We live in a culture that regards happiness as the human norm and suffering as the aberration. In opposing this paradigm, Judaism is coun-tercultural, reminding us that suffering is a built-in feature of everyone's life. Suffering is no mitzvah, and we do not actively search for it, but nei-ther can we escape or avoid it; suffering is as constituent a part of our human reality as love and joy.

While Judaism does not foresee the elimination of suffering as a pos-sibility in our world, it does provide us with institutions and structures for meliorating suffering. Eric Cassell has written that "recovery from suf-fering involved borrowing the strength of others as though persons who have lost parts of themselves can be sustained by the personhood of oth-ers until their own recovers."[16] Synagogues can serve as communities of strength for the sufferer and for his or her caregiver. In the synagogue one can find co-sufferers and fellow caregivers who can succor us with an emotional identification that only they can have. Through the syna-gogue, despite our suffering, we can experience that traditional acclama-tion at the end of the reading of a book of Torah: "Be strong, be strong, and strengthen one another."

Judaism also furnishes us with prayers to cope with our suffering. Healing services, which join together in worship all those who are ill or hurting, have become common in most synagogues. Healing services have deep roots in Jewish liturgy, which reach back to the *Mi Shebeirach* blessing of the Torah service and the blessing for health in the *Amidah*. In both these blessings, individualized prayers for the recovery of the sick and the suffering are rendered. The idea of praying for health predates even these ancient blessings. Moses himself called out a prayer for his sis-ter's restoration to wholeness: "*El na r'fa na lah*—O God, please heal her!" (Numbers 12:13). In later times, many Jews found the sustenance to cope with their suffering by reciting psalms, especially Psalms 20, 23, 30, 121, 130, and 150. The central message of the psalms is one of hope, and reading them in any language can bring strength to the sufferer and his or her caregiver.

Prayer allows us to transcend the present moment and to locate ourselves in a context larger than our immediate suffering. Prayer enables us to go beyond the isolation created by our pain and to place our suffering in a Jewish framework that is shared by our community. Prayer points to the transpersonal and collective dimension of our suffering, causing us to see it as part and parcel of other people's suffering. Prayer thus pushes us beyond ourselves into empathy with the suffering of others.

A third practice, in addition to synagogue participation and prayer, particularly well suited for caregivers of those in pain, is the old-new ritual of *hitbod'dut*. *Hitbod'dut* refers to the kabbalistic form of meditation that literally means self-isolation. Rabbi Nachman of Bratzlav (1772–1810) was a master of *hitbod'dut*, and for him it meant a daily period of aloneness. He wrote, "Set aside an hour or more each day to meditate, in the fields or in a room, pouring out your thoughts to God."[17] In our day, *hitbod'dut* often takes the shape of quiet walks or extended periods of sitting in which the individual turns inward and articulates to God his or her deepest needs and fears. Through *hitbod'dut* one can find a personal closeness to God that often eludes us in formal prayer services and that can confer upon us renewal and strength.

Conclusion

What we human beings fear most in this world is chaos. The most awesome terror we face is meaninglessness. Suffering threatens us with this. Suffering disorients us to the world, shatters our easy routines, and makes a mockery of our cherished beliefs. Suffering portends the extinction of our selves and the end to any meaning we might attach to ourselves, our contributions to the world, and our relationships. Suffering jeopardizes our every claim to self-worth.

Through belief, practice, and sacred text, Judaism offers us hope in transcendence. Our tradition acknowledges the truth of suffering but does not seek to locate meaning in it; rather, Judaism provides us with the tools to go beyond it morally, ritually, and theologically. Let us neither deny nor rejoice in suffering; let us use it to draw closer to our true selves, to other people, and to our God.

When the Time Came

<hr>

        ☙ ❧

Dr. James Soffer

I started to notice her speech was different. There seemed to be a slight slur. Our semi-weekly phone conversations were otherwise the same as usual: "What have you been doing, how are you feeling, what are the kids up to?" As the weeks progressed, though, and the slur continued, I asked my sister, Trish, if she had noticed. "Is mom hitting the bottle [she never did before]? Could it be a mini-stroke?"

About a year before, I had asked my mother if she had noticed her altered speech. She had noticed it, but at the time she was undergoing extensive periodontal and reconstructive dentistry, so the likelihood existed that it was related to that. Aside from her speech difficulties, she felt the same as usual, which wasn't so good anyway. She had been in general good health, but rarely felt very well. For about thirty years she had suffered from fatigue syndrome, as a result of a tropical illness contracted while on a cruise. Due to this, she spent an extraordinary amount of time resting, in order to have energy to do anything. And she loved to do things. Playing cards was her passion—she played a few times a week. She also loved to dance. Another passion of hers was health and nutrition. Because conventional remedies had been unable to cure her chronic fatigue, she became obsessed with excellent nutrition and turned to homeopathic and herbal remedies.

Her dental work was now completed, but her speech continued to deteriorate. She thought the dentist must have damaged some nerves or administered too much anesthesia. As a dentist myself, I knew that was unlikely. Meanwhile, blood chemistry and hair analysis revealed enormous levels of mercury in her body. Mercury, a heavy metal, could cause the neurological effects that she was experiencing.

She began detoxification treatments at a homeopathic clinic—a series of injections and questionable treatment at a large fee. Trish began her own research and arrived at the possible diagnosis that I hadn't wished to suggest. I had suspected ALS, but I couldn't even say the words. Since I knew there was no successful treatment, I did not discourage any treatment that gave my mother hope. In early December, my mother was referred to neurologists, who confirmed mercury poisoning, but also indicated that there might be another contributing diagnosis.

For the winter vacation, Mom joined my family in Cancún. We knew that this might be the last time we would be together and were looking forward to spending a wonderful week. Although my mother required her periods of rest, she always seemed to have plenty of energy to shop the native markets. Mealtimes were difficult, however, and sitting by her was painful as she constantly choked on her meals. Her speech was slow and slurred, and difficult to understand, but we were still able to converse with her. The week we spent there will be a lasting memory, especially for my sons.

Upon returning to Florida, Mom became an outpatient at the Miami Parkinson Institute, the local center for diagnosis and treatment for ALS. The facilities were limited, but the doctors were knowledgeable and as helpful as my mother would allow. The diagnosis was confirmed to be ALS. Mom made it clear that she would not linger when the end was imminent, would not go to a nursing home, and would not allow a feeding tube to be placed, as it would only prolong the agony.

Beginning in the fall, Trish and I had begun a monthly, then biweekly, then weekly commute, sometimes with each other, sometimes alone. Once Trish took her whole family to say a last good-bye. At each visit Mom was a bit thinner and a bit weaker, but still tried to maintain some social activities. On Saturdays we often went to the flea market, and in the evening we always went out for dinner, as difficult as it was. As time went on, she would no longer speak on the phone, except to Trish and me, and a few select friends. Her card games were reduced to once a week, to minimize embarrassment. We were not permitted to tell anyone the diagnosis or the true reason for her inability to speak.

May 8 of that year was Mother's Day, and Trish and I had gone to be with her for the weekend. Mom seemed more depressed and weaker than before. The weather, however, was beautiful, and Trish and I went to the beach. This time my mother joined us and even went into the ocean with us for the first time in maybe forty years. The sight of her emaciated body in a bathing suit was shocking. I hadn't realized how thin she had become. Her attempts at eating and drinking were becoming futile. It was clear that any swallowing would soon be an impossibility. We returned home on Sunday knowing that there wouldn't be many more trips.

On a Tuesday, Trish said Mom was failing and that she would return to Florida the next day. I told her to let me know how Mom was and if she needed me. When she arrived, Mom was very weak, spent most of the time sleeping, and could no longer swallow. By the time I arrived, it was clear that the end was coming. We called hospice, who gave us medications to keep Mom comfortable and provided all of us with support for what would be the most difficult next five days. During that time, we rarely left the bedroom. We stayed with Mom, talking, crying, wetting her lips, stroking her hand or forehead, watching her breathing become shallower and slower.

There were few decisions for us to make at that point; Mom and the circumstances dictated our course. We took care of our mother and honored her wish for a peaceful passing. We relied upon each other for the strength to keep from falling apart. Trish said I was her hero, but I felt she was mine.

I could never imagine how I would handle the death of my parents. I wouldn't allow myself to even think about it, but when the time came, I did what I had to. There was no choice.

The Torah commands that we honor and obey our mother and father. We fulfilled the mitzvah. Mom died peacefully on May 19, 1998.

❧

Accepting Death:
The Caregiver's Dilemma

RABBI W. GUNTHER PLAUT

While in some ancient cultures death was believed to be a separate force, Jewish tradition saw it as an ineluctable aspect of all existence. The Tree of Life remains inaccessible to us; we are dust, and to dust we return (Genesis 2:7; 3:19; Job 10:9). A second-century tale reports that Rabbi Meir had a Torah manuscript in which the usual description of God's creation as *tov m'od*, "very good," read *tov mot*, "death is good" (*B'reishit Rabbah* 9:5). Without death, life as we know it would be impossible. But before we can appreciate how Rabbi Meir could have said this, we have to abandon the contemporary belief that death is not inevitable. While for us it has the status of abnormality, for the ancients life and death were a normal sequence.

Biblical records tell us of farewells in down-to-earth tones, each describing a realistic parting that has finality written all over it. Of Isaac we read that when he was old he said to his elder son Esau: "I am old now, and I do not know how soon I will die. . . . Prepare a dish that I like, so that [after I eat it] I may give you my heartfelt blessing before I die" (Genesis 27:2, 4).

Jacob's blessing of his children is reported as a vision of the future: "So Jacob called his twelve sons together and said: 'Assemble so that I may tell you what lies ahead for you in days to come'" (Genesis 49:1). The most unsentimental good-bye recorded in the Bible is King David's parting words to his son Solomon: "I am about to go the way of all flesh, so be strong and show yourself a man." He then proceeded to instruct him to take revenge on Joab son of Zeruiah for having killed two of Israel's commanders and to do the same to Shimei son of Gera, who had insulted David, but to honor Barzillai the Gileadite because he had saved him from his pursuers. Not a tinge of sentimental parting (I Kings 2:1–10).

What all these good-byes have in common is an unquestioned acceptance of death as a natural event. That does not mean that loved ones who were left behind did not mourn—of Abraham it is expressly said that he bewailed his wife's departure from this earth (Genesis 23:2). Tears came to mourners then as they come now, but the acceptance of death as a reality of existence was fundamentally different. They dealt with it openly and straightforwardly, while we tend to hide or even deny it.

Why then can't we react to death as the ancients did? Because we believe in the unlimited power of science to overcome all obstacles, from intergalactic travel to analyzing and altering genes. Average longevity is steadily increasing, so why not presume that we can extend it forever? We continue to look for the right doctor, the miraculous medicine, or whatever it is that promises to turn the Angel of Death away—temporarily at least, but maybe even indefinitely.

An appreciation that death is natural is understandably difficult when the dying are those close to us. The beliefs we may have held about death and dying are often useless when it comes to our own loved ones. We don't want to part from them, and many of us hope that the final farewell is not final at all. Though Jewish tradition offers no such promise, we hope that perchance we may see one another again—somewhere, somehow. The old idea of God's reviving the dead is messianic imagery, and the prayer asking God to admit the deceased to paradisiacal existence[1] is purposefully undefined. We Jews are not taught to expect the dead to change into angelic spirits.

Our reluctance to face death squarely often robs the dying of the opportunity to depart with peace and dignity. Some years ago a close friend of mine lay on his deathbed. I pleaded with the family to let me talk to him of death, for I was sure that such openness would make it possible for him to bless his children and have a measure of closure. But the immediate family rejected the idea, claiming that their loved one would be unable to confront reality. "Better he should go in ignorance," they said. "There will be less heartache all around."

Fortunately, medical and psychological practitioners no longer believe that ignoring the reality of death is the best approach. While not everyone reacts in the same fashion, and some who are dying may indeed be unable to face the truth about their prospects, most will be glad to be relieved of the charade that is being played. They likely know that they are about to die and that the family also knows. Repeated assurances that they are "doing fine" mean that their dying occurs in a vacuum created by denial. We should be given a chance to end our earthly existence with honesty rather than with deception, however well motivated.

My wife Elizabeth and I often discussed these matters and agreed that we would face approaching death as openly as possible. As we climbed the ladder of aging we drew up mutual powers of attorney for personal care, or living wills. The documents expressed our desire not to be kept artificially alive when such procedure could not advance recovery. But neither of us anticipated what happened shortly after the millennium took its bow. Elizabeth suffered a stroke and was rushed to the hospital. After a few days she made good progress: her mind was unaffected, her speech returned fairly well, and we waited for her application to a rehabilitation hospital to be approved. But before that could happen she had another series of strokes, this time dreadfully extensive. She became almost totally paralyzed and can now only beat the lower part of one arm up and down, a motion that has become her main avenue of expressing her feelings. Her eyes are open, but she cannot speak. I do not know whether she knows me, her husband of sixty-two years, or whom or what she knows. I believe she is unaware of her condition, for she appears quite comfortable, having the best of care in a splendid hospital that is adept at caring for patients like her. A turnaround is deemed unlikely by the experts, who tell me that her condition may remain unchanged for years. She lives in a world that is inaccessible to others. I visit her every day and tell myself that I must accept the situation as it is, but often leave depressed and struggle to keep my mental balance.

I suffer the caregiver's ultimate dilemma: I do not know what to hope and pray for. That cognition return to her, which most likely would thrust her into deep depression? I dare not impose upon her my own sense of what a meaningful quality of life would be. The *Mi Shebeirach* that is sung in the synagogue speaks in general tones of healing body and spirit, and I chant the words with all my heart and mind. Meanwhile, she no doubt has some sort of inner existence. She cries when she is uncomfortable, and her arm beats up and down when I kiss her or when she hears a melody she likes. Neurologists are just as ignorant about the workings of her brain as I am.

The hospital authorities have asked to know whether Elizabeth had expressed any wishes about being kept alive. The statement we drew up fits what the doctors call "DNR"—meaning "do not resuscitate and keep alive artificially." In medical practice this applies to something like cardiac arrest. But if, for instance, the patient has pneumonia, the hospital will administer antibiotics as usual and will treat every other untoward development in the spirit of the Hippocratic oath.

Some well-meaning friends say that she'd be better off if she were to die peacefully. But despite my acceptance of death, that is something I cannot and will not pray for. Judaism deems life itself to be a sacred gift. It does not permit me to impose upon her my values of what may be judged to be a "worthwhile life." I have said the *Vidui*, the traditional deathbed confession for a few of my parishioners. Would I be able to say the words for my wife, who could not repeat them as tradition suggests? I wonder.[2] As long as she is alive I nurture some hope of healing, however little it may be.

"Immortality of the soul" is the term most often attached to the belief that we survive death in some fashion. While the Bible does not dwell on the subject, the Rabbis, under the influence of Plato and his Jewish counterpart Philo, opted for the hope that something of us survives our earthly demise. Though the flesh decays, the soul ascends toward heaven or descends toward *Geihinom*, the place of permanent perdition. A traditional argument for this tradition maintains that God has created us and our faculties with a certain purpose and has instilled within us the yearning for immortality. This very fact is seen as pointing to its reality. The traditional prayer book praises God as *m'chayei hameitim*, "who revives the dead," while *Gates of Prayer*, the Reform *siddur*, generally substitutes for it a neutral *m'chayei hakol*, "the Source of life."

I believe that the best in us will be immortal. How much and in what fashion I do not and cannot know. I find immortality of the soul a good possibility, but I do not strive to earn it. Will it be a conscious personal existence as it is now? Will I again meet my late brother, my parents, and my departed friends? I for one do not believe this—but if I am wrong, so much the better. Meanwhile I live my life the best I can and leave the rest to God.[3]

Death is and will remain a mystery. Its modern denial leads us into blind alleys and renders us helpless when we are facing the end. Accepting death as a reality that befalls all creatures makes us who are caregivers comrades with the dying in the fight for meaning and dignity. Saying goodbye with love, compassion, and sharing our faith may strengthen us and give tranquility to the one who is about to leave us.

Letting the Cycle of Life Do Its Work:
The Miracle of Death

_____

☙ ❧

Rabbi Hara E. Person

I no longer remember if it took three days, four days, or a full week. There is a great deal I don't remember about those last days. But I do remember being called by my mother on her cell phone to go over to the hospital and sit with my grandmother, who had suddenly gotten much worse. The hospital staff weren't sure she would make it through the night.

My parents rushed back to the city from their trip upstate, and in the meantime, I went over to the hospital. My grandmother lay in her bed, small and lost among the white bedcovers. An oxygen mask was over her mouth, and her chest rose and fell rhythmically, but with great effort. Her watery blue eyes were wide open, but she didn't seem to see anyone, or anything.

I sat down next to her and spoke. I asked her how she was feeling and if she needed me to do anything for her. There was no reaction. I held her hand in mine and stroked her forehead. I talked to her, telling stories about my children, and reassured her, over and over, that everything was okay. The night wore on as I waited for my mother to arrive. My grandmother continued to breathe in and out, in and out, laboriously.

It was another attack of pneumonia, which my grandmother had caught repeatedly throughout the last three years. Each time she would get sicker than I thought someone could get and still survive, more confused and disoriented than before, until the antibiotics would bring her back to a semi-lucid state. So many times she had asked to die, so many times she had fought medication and refused IVs. But in the end she was always treated, even when it meant tying her with restraints, and being released back to the nursing home.

I believed that my grandmother wanted to die. She had always been a proud, strong, independent woman, and now she was reduced to something she had always despised. She was angry and depressed and took out her anger on those closest to her. While I loved her and wanted her to live and be well, I could also understand her wish to die. Her life, for all intents and purposes, was over. There were times, during our many repeated emergency room visits, that I too got angry. Angry that she was being kept alive when she clearly didn't want to live any longer. Angry that medical technology existed to keep her body alive when her brain was gone. Angry that she could live when the essence of whom she had been had departed some time ago. Angry at myself for not being able to value who she now was, versus who she had been before. Angry that the grandmother I loved had been stolen from us, and from herself. Not to treat her with antibiotics seemed clearly cruel and unethical. Yet for all that I valued the miracle that is human life, I couldn't figure out how to accept that her life was still a life worth living. How could God want someone to keep living like that? What was the point of keeping her alive? And then angry at myself for not being able to understand.

This time was different. Her illness had reached a new point. She was no longer able to fight or argue or state her wishes. Over the next few days and nights, we kept vigil at my grandmother's bedside. My sister and I took turns spelling my mother. The hospital staff announced that this time was for real. She was dying. And we had agreed that she shouldn't die alone, not only because it wouldn't be right Jewishly, but because we could do no less for someone we loved. So the bleak, hot, steamy hospital room became our temporary familial landscape. We talked to her, we read to her, we told her stories. One late night I recited psalms and read the *Vidui*, and another night my husband sang her favorite song, "Shaina Di Lavuneh," into her ear. As I sat next to her and rubbed her hand, I repeated words of reassurance to let her know that it was okay to leave us, that we would be okay, and that she would be okay as well. I told her that if she wanted to keep fighting, that was great, but that if she was ready to let go, we were ready to let her go. Sometimes my grandmother's eyebrows would rise, as if she could hear us. But at some point over those few days, her eyes closed for good and her face grew more relaxed. Her breathing grew shallower, but steadier. I hadn't noticed it happening, but the change was suddenly clear.

I was grateful that my mother seemed ready to accept that it was time to let her go. It was not easy to give up hope and accept that death had arrived. There was nothing we could do any longer to keep death from the doorway; all we could do at that point was choose how long, drawn out, and technologically controlled the dying process would be. It took several days and many long, painful discussions, but in the end my mother chose to honor the wishes my grandmother had made while she was still healthy about not wanting any extraordinary measures taken to extend her life. Once we made that decision as a family and went through the bureaucratic hoops to make sure that the hospital wouldn't act against our wishes, a feeling of holiness and peace pervaded that hospital room. The choice to let the cycle of life do its work, instead of artificially prolonging life, was a great relief. Harsh lights were dimmed. Beeping machines were stilled. The doctors were instructed to simply make my grandmother as comfortable as possible.

Having made the decision to refuse a feeding tube, respirator, and all the other means of artificially sustaining life, we were able to stop pretending that my grandmother might suddenly recover and revert back to the dynamo she used to be. We were able to accept that there was only so much we could do to guide God's hand and that, in the end, death is as much of a miracle as birth. Our roles changed from being advocates for my grandmother's life to being midwives to her death. In the dimmed lights of that sterile hospital room, the work of dying was taking place, a process no less holy than the labor of living. Letting my grandmother float into death felt like the most respectful way to allow her to leave this world, not angry and fighting, but gently ushered out by those who loved her.

I no longer remember whether it took three days or a week. Late one night I kissed my grandmother good-bye and left my mother in the hospital for the night shift. My grandmother died early the next morning, with her daughter at her side, holding her hand. After three and half years of watching my grandmother suffer and disintegrate, we were able to mourn and grieve the woman she had been. I was thankful for the miracle of life that had been my grandmother and thankful for the miracle of a peaceful death that had been granted her.

ᗧᕮᗩ

Notes

⊂℥ ℬ⊃

Introduction: Celebrating the Art of Caregiving

1. Susan Bortz, correspondence, 2000.

Caring for Our Parents, Caring for Ourselves: A Jewish Perspective

1. Moses Maimonides, *Mishneh Torah*, Hilchot De'ot, 4:1.
2. Moses Maimonides, *The Preservation of Youth: Essays on Health*, trans. Hirsch L. Gordon (New York: The Wisdom Library, 1958), 47.
3. Hayim Halevy Donin, *To Be a Jew* (New York: Basic Books, 1972), 60.
4. Benjamin Blech, *Understanding Judaism: The Basics of Deed and Creed* (Northvale, N.J.: Jason Aronson, 1992), 12.

Caring for Our Parents by Making Decisions Together

1. Betty Friedan, *The Fountain of Age* (New York: Simon & Schuster, 1993), 13.
2. See BT *Kiddushin* 32b; Maimonides' *Code*, The Laws Regarding *Talmud Torah*, 6:9; and *Sefer HaChinuch*, Mitzvah No. 257.
3. Mark H. Beers and Stephen K. Urice, *Aging in Good Health: A Complete Essential Medical Guide for Older Men and Women and Their Families* (New York: Pocket Books, 1992), 46.
4. Robert Butler and Myrna Lewis, *Aging and Mental Health* (New York: New American Library, 1983), 111.
5. Beers and Urice, *Aging in Good Health* (New York: Pocket Books, 1992), 5.

6. Solomon Ganzfried, *Code of Jewish Law: Kitzur Shulchan Aruch* (New York: Hebrew Publishing Company, 1963), 4:89.

7. There are two types of nursing homes. A skilled nursing facility provides twenty-four-hour care, staffed with medically qualified persons. The residential care facilities are places where care is provided but residents are in need of less medical care.

8. Lee Olitzky. *Handmaker Elder Care Handbook: A Resource Guide for Those Providing Support and Care to Elders* (Tucson, Ariz.: Handmaker Management Enterprises, 1997).

9. Sharon Strassfeld and Kathy Green, *The Jewish Family Book* (New York: Bantom Books, 1976), 389.

10. See Jack Riemer and Nathaniel Stampfer's *So That Your Values Live On – Ethical Wills and How to Prepare Them* (Vermont: Jewish Lights Publishing, 1991).

11. Olitzky, *Handmaker Elder Care Handbook*, 12–14.

12. For greater elaboration on this subject, see Butler and Lewis, *Aging and Mental Health*, 11–15.

13. Louis I. Newman, *Hasidic Anthology* (New York: Schocken Books, 1972), 6.

Jewish Values and Sociopsychological Perspectives on Aging

1. Cf. *Jewish Encyclopedia*, s.v. "Age, Old," for original sources.

2. Ibid.

3. Cf. David Riesman, *The Lonely Crowd* (New Haven: Yale University Press, 1950).

4. Erik H. Erikson, *Childhood and Society* (New York: W.W. Norton & Co., 1950), 219–34.

5. Robert J. Havighurst, *Human Development and Education* (New York: Longmans Green, 1953).

6. Maimonides, *Mishneh Torah, Hilchot Deot*.

7. *Pirkei Avot*: 5:21.

8. *Jewish Encyclopedia*, s.v. "Ages of Man in Jewish Literature, The Seven."

9. Erikson, *Childhood and Society*.

10. Joseph Campbell, *The Hero with a Thousand Faces* (New York: Meridian Books, 1956), 30.

11. Ibid.

12. John R. Silber, "The Pollution of Time," *The Center Magazine* 4, no. 5 (September-October 1971).

13. Ibid.

14. Ibid.

15. Seymour L. Halleck, "What Adults Have Against Children," *The Enquirer Magazine*, Cincinnati, February 6, 1972, p. 35, reprinted from the *I B M Think Magazine*, November-December 1970.

16. Sebastian de Grazia, *Of Time, Work, and Leisure* (New York: Twentieth Century Fund, 1962), 153.

17. Margaret Mead, *Culture and Commitment* (New York: Natural History Press, 1970).

18. Ibid.

19. BT *Sotah* 49b.

20. *Tosefta Avodah Zarah* 1:19.

21. Simone de Beauvoir, *The Coming of Age*, trans. Patrick O'Brian (New York: Warner Publications, 1973), 807.

22. Zena Smith Blau, *Old Age in a Changing Society* (New York: Watts, 1973).

23. Philip Slater, *The Pursuit of Loneliness: American Culture at the Breaking Point* (Boston: Beacon Press, 1970), 80.

24. De Beauvoir, *Coming of Age*, 666.

25. Herbert Marcuse, *Eros and Civilization* (New York: Vintage Books, 1955), 66.

26. Ibid.

27. Ibid.

28. Cf. the essay by Rabbi Norman Lamm on "Ethics and Leisure" in his *Faith and Doubt* (New York: Ktav Publishing Company, 1971), 187–209.

29. Ibid.

30. Maimonides, *Mishneh Torah, Hilchot M'lachim*, 12:4 ff.

Spiritual Aging

1. Mary Bray Pipher, *Another Country: Navigating the Emotional Terrain of Our Elders* (New York: Riverhead Books, 2000).

2. Abraham Joshua Heschel, *The Sabbath* (New York: Farrar, Straus, and Giroux, 1951), 4.

Five Women Spanning Four Generations

1. The *Shechinah*, in Jewish tradition, is God's Divine Presence in the feminine form.

2. This portion of the Torah is known as the Holiness Code. Scholars point to the connection to the Ten Commandments. The fact that honoring one's parents is in the Decalogue and holding one's parents in awe is in the Holiness Code points to the weight the Torah places in showing honor and awe to one's parents.

3. Rashi to Leviticus 19:3.

4. I learned this concept from Dr. Ruth Harriet Jacobs when I took a course called "Aging: Reengaging in Later Life" at Boston University. She was one of the finest teachers I have ever had.

5. *z"l* represent the Hebrew words *Zichrono(ah) livrachah*, "May his (her) memory be for a blessing." These initials written after someone's name is an indication that the person has died. The expression *Zichrono(ah) livrachah*; "May his (her) memory be for a blessing," reminds the living that our beloved dead leave a precious memory that serves to bring blessing.

Beyond Guilt: What We Owe Our Aging Parents— A Perspective from Tradition

1. My stepfather, Fred Marcus, *z"l*, died six months after this essay was written. It is respectfully dedicated in his memory.

2. For a very useful analysis of caregiving today and the gap between this reality and the widespread perception that the current generation is caring for elders less assiduously than our forebears, see Elaine M. Brody, "Parent Care as a Normative Family Stress," *The Gerontologist* 25, no. 1 (1985): 19–29.

3. A version of this story is found in *Yiddish Folktales*, ed. Beatrice Silverman Weinreich (New York: Pantheon Books, 1988). It dates to the 17th or 18th century, and is cited by Glückel of Hameln in her memoir.

4. The literal translation of the verse, "A man shall revere his mother and his father," has been rendered here in a more inclusive manner.

5. See, for example, BT *Kiddushin* 32a, and compare JT *Kiddushin* 1:7 and Maimonides' *Mishneh Torah, Hilchot Mamrim* 6:3.

6. Danny Siegel, "The *Mitzvah* of Bringing Out the Beauty in Our Elders' Faces," in *A Heart of Wisdom: Making the Jewish Journey from Midlife through the Elder Years*, ed. Susan Berrin (Woodstock, Vt.: Jewish Lights Publishing, 1997), 51.

7. William Thomas, *Life Worth Living: How Someone You Love Can Still Enjoy Life in a Nursing Home—The Eden Alternative in Action* (Acton, Mass.: VanderWyk and Burnham, 1996).

8. Maimonides, *Mishneh Torah, Hilchot Ishut* 13:14. This text conveys different approaches for husbands and wives, reflecting marital and gender roles of the era in which it was written

9. This narrative and other case examples are composites of actual cases, with details changed to protect the confidentiality of the individuals described in them.

10. See, for example, BT *Kiddushin* 31a–32a.

11. Maimonides, *Mishneh Torah, Hilchot Mamrim* 6:10.

12. Those who work in nursing homes often find that families care assiduously for relatives with dementia, avoiding placement until they are absolutely overwhelmed. Often, a parent's becoming incontinent will be the "last straw" event that leads to placement, as neither parents nor their children want toileting to be part of their relationship.

13. *Sefer Chasidim* 343:257.

14. Maimonides, *Mishneh Torah, Hilchot Mamrim* 6:8–9.

15. *Shulchan Aruch* 240:18.

Honor Your Father and Mother: Caregiving as a Halachic Responsibility

1. This is not likely to be a result of any lack of awareness of growth in the relationship as a child moves from the total dependency of infancy to the independence of adulthood; the discussion of the Babylon Talmud follows directly on a discussion of parental obligations to their young children (BT *Kiddushin* 31b–32a).

This emphasis of the halachic corpus on the relationship between adult children and their parents is revealed only when one traces the actual discussions of this issue in the major collections of the responsa literature. The largest group of discussions by far in the more recent responsa deal with the question of how to continue honoring one's parents after they have passed away. They indicate that adults are asking the halachic questions; that honoring their parents has been a significant expression of their religiosity, built up over a lifetime relationship; and that to discontinue the mitzvah because of death seems unnatural to them, deepening their sense of loss. This issue is particularly important for children who have lost parents in the Holocaust.

2. Primary loci of these discussions include *M'Chilta D'Rabbi Yishmael, Yitro, D'bachodesh* 8; *Sifra K'doshim* 1; BT *Kiddushin* 31b; JT *Pei-ah* 1:1; JT *Kiddushin* 1:7.

3. *Mishnah Pei-ah* 1:1.

4. For a summary discussion of this issue, see Louis Novick, in "Workshop: Family Responsibility to the Elderly," in *Aging in the Jewish World: Continuity and Change*, Second International Symposium, Jerusalem, July 1989, ed. Shimon Bergman and Jack Habib (Jerusalem: Magnes Press, 1992), 200–201. See also Walter Jacob, *Contemporary American Reform Responsa* (New York: Central Conference of American Rabbis, 1987), YD 26, pp. 44–45.

5. Gerald Blidstein, *Honor Thy Father and Mother: Filial Responsibility in Jewish Law and Ethics* (New York: Ktav, 1975), 39.

6. Maimonides, *Mishneh Torah, Hilchot Mamrim* 6:1.

7. Michael Chernick phrases this slightly differently, pointing out that the Talmud's removal of the emotional level from this discussion is related to the impossibility of legislating emotions as opposed to easily dictated actions. Although an accurate observation, this seems to me to limit the possible dimensions in which one can understand filial obligations. See his "Who Pays? The Talmudic Approach to Filial Responsibility," *The Journal of Aging of Judaism* 1 (1987): 111–12, also reproduced in this volume.

Steven Carr Reuben similarly misses the beauty of this elevation of the commandment. He comments that the rabbinic fear of abandonment in old age at a time of physical decline and increasing inability to be self-sufficient led the Rabbis to develop a "strong set of injunctions and social mores that upheld the significance of honoring one's parents as being equal to if not greater than honoring God Himself. For the sake of survival, it was necessary for all to recognize the debilitating effects that old age had upon the individual, and to legislate either legally, socially, or both to protect the aged from the ravages of their human condition" ("Old Age: Appearance and Reality," *Journal of Psychology and Judaism* 16 [1992]: 186). Given the rather minimal attention paid to this commandment in the rabbinic corpus, specifically as it applies to the debilities of very old age, and given that it is only with recent demographic and medical shifts that old age and extended disability have become a common factor of human experience, Reuben has significantly overstated his case and given an unnecessarily cynical reading to the rabbinic pronouncements.

8. As reported in James A. Thorson, *Aging in a Changing Society* (Belmont, Calif.: Wadsworth Publishing Company, 1995), 405.

9. Ibid., 63, 72.

10. See Tamara K. Hareven, "Family and Generational Relations in the Later Years: A Historical Perspective," *Generations* (Summer 1992), 9–10.

11. Elaine M. Brody, "Parent Care as a Normative Family Stress," *The Gerontologist* 25 (1985): 23.

12. Blidstein, *Honor,* 8–19, presents a sophisticated survey of the sources from the Bible to the *Acharonim*.

13. See, for example, Jane English, "What Do Grown Children Owe Their Parents?" in *Aging and Ethics: Philosophical Problems in Gerontology*, ed. Nancy S. Jecker, (Totowa, N.J.: Humana Press, 1992); reports from *Philosophical and Legal Reflections on Parenthood* (New York: Oxford University Press, 1979), 147–54.

14. Hareven, "Family," 9, 12.

15. Exemplified most dramatically in the statement of Rabbi Yochanan, who was orphaned from birth, "Happy is the person who has no parents," to which Rashi comments, "For it is impossible to honor them to the degree necessary, and one is consequently punished because of them" (BT *Kiddushin* 31b).

16. See, especially, Brody, "Patient Care," 20–25.

17. Ibid., 21.

18. See Emeric Deutsch, "Changes in Relations within Jewish Families and Consequences for the Elderly," in *Aging in the Jewish World: Continuity and Change*, Second International Symposium, Jerusalem, 1989 (Jerusalem: Magnes Press, 1992), 153.

Beyond the few relevant pages in Blidstein's volume, substantive discussions of our issue can be found in the presentations of Rabbi Reuven P. Bulka and Rabbi Barry Freundel for *The Orthodox Roundtable*, Heshvan/Kislev 5754, entitled, respectively, "Honoring Parents—The Extents and the Limits" and "The Care of Elderly Parents"; and Freundel's article "Halakhah and the Nursing Home Dilemma," *Proceedings of the Association of Orthodox Jewish Scientists* (1990): 85–106; Levi Meier, "Filial Responsibility to the Senile Parent: A Jewish Perspective," in *Spiritual Well-Being of the Elderly*, ed. James A. Thorson and Thomas C. Cook, Jr. (Springfield, Ill.: Charles C. Thomas, Publisher, 1980), 161–68; and Immanuel Jakobovits, "Ethical Guidelines for an Aging Jewish World," *International Forum* IF-9-86 (Jerusalem: J.D.C., Brookdale Institute of Gerontology and Adult Human Development in Israel, 1985). Neither Freundel nor I have located any further halachic discussion of our question.

19. Maimonides, *Mishneh Torah, Hilchot Mamrim* 6:7.

20. Ibid., 6:8.

21. Ibid., 6:9.

22. This point relates to the idea of sanctity of the Land of Israel, a major polemical point among third-century Palestinian Rabbis in their working to keep the center of authority of Judaism within the Land. See Isaiah Gafni's book on the subject.

23. BT *Kiddushin* 31b.

24. R. David in Zimra (Radbaz), commenting on Maimonides (see below), points out that these inappropriate demands were also ones she could not make of a stranger.

25. Maimonides, *Mishneh Torah, Hilchot Mamrim* 6:10.

26. Maimonides, *Yoreh Dei-ah* 240:10.

27. Others have discussed many of the issues raised here, see particularly Barry Freundel, "Halakhah and the Nursing Home Dilemma,"

Proceedings of the Association of Orthodox Jewish Scientists (1990), 85–106; Immanuel Jakobovits, "Ethical Guidelines for an Aging Jewish World," *International Forum*, F-9-86 (Jerusalem: J.D.C., Brookdale Institute of Gerontology and Adult Human Development in Israel, 1985); Rabbi Reuven P. Bulka, "Honoring Parents—The Extents and the Limits," *The Orthodox Roundtable* (Heshvan/Kislev 5754). The lack of discussion of these issues in the Hebrew responsa literature is surprising.

28. On this issue, see the *Tzitz Eliezer*, vol. 12, no. 59.

29. Maimonides, *Mishneh Torah, Hilchot Mamrim* 6:6; *Yoreh Dei-ah* 240:17.

30. Brody, "Patient Care," 21.

31. We cannot establish from the texts available, though, how many daughters-in-law actually performed many of the tasks that the halachah assigned to their husbands; nor can we establish how many sons actually let their sisters carry the burden. Of course, much of the answer lies in whether a specific community expected sons or daughters to take up residence with or near their parents.

32. Maimonides, *Yoreh Dei-ah* 240:5. The only limitation on this is that one need not impoverish oneself to the point that one lacks sufficient food for a single day. At that point, one's own livelihood takes priority.

33. Brody, "Patient Care," 25.

34. This is analogous to the contemporary concern that the elderly carefully prepare for the disposition of their property and explicitly state their wishes about difficult health-care decisions.

A Jewish Way of Thinking about Nursing Homes

1. For a full discussion of these ideas, see Dennis Sylva, *Psalms and the Transformation of Stress: Poetic-Communal Interpretation and the Family*, Louvain Theological & Pastoral Monographs 16 (Louvain, Belgium: Peeters Press, 1993), chap. 9.

2. Virginia Morris, *How to Care for Aging Parents* (New York: Workman Publishing, 1996), 209.

3. Ruth Langer, "Honor Your Father and Mother: Caregiving as a Halachic Responsibility," in *Aging and the Aged in Jewish Law: Essays and Responsa*, ed. Walter Jacob and Moshe Zemer (Pittsburgh and Tel Aviv: Freehof Institute of Progressive Halakhah, 1998), 22, also reproduced in this volume.

4. Solomon B. Freehof, *New Reform Responsa* (Cincinnati: Hebrew Union College Press, 1980), chap. 22.

5. Isserles's gloss to *Yoreh Dei-ah* 240:4.

6. Freehof, *New Reform Responsa*, 95.

7. Maimonides, *Mishneh Torah, Hilchot Mamrim* 6:10.

8. Langer, "Honor," 33, 38.

9. W. Carole Chenitz, "Entry into a Nursing Home as Status Passage: A Theory to Guide Nursing Practice," *Geriatric Nursing*, March/April 1983, 92.

10. Ibid., 96.

11. Ibid., 94.

12. See Walter Brueggemann's *The Message of the Psalms* (Minneapolis: Augsburg Publishing House, 1984), in which he argues that the Book of Psalms is organized around three themes: poems of orientation, poems of disorientation, and poems of new orientation.

13. Marge Pelzmann, *Reducing Stress When Relocating Older People*, a brochure describing the research of Michael E. Hunt, Arch. D., School of Family Resources and Consumer Sciences, University of Wisconsin–Madison; the research was funded by the AARP Andrus Foundation of Washington, D.C., through the Institute on Aging, University of Wisconsin–Madison. The University of Michigan study, cited in the brochure, was the basis of Hunt's research.

14. Susan Grossman, "Tahanun: More than Mere 'Supplication,'" *Sh'ma: A Journal of Jewish Responsibility* 22/436 (4 September 1992): 126–27.

15. We can encourage, and try to enable, an older adult to be verbally expressive and resilient, but we need to be realistic in our goals if these are not qualities the older person already possesses. At the same time, the cultivation of this ancient survival strategy is a worthy goal in the formulation of Jewish history curricula for children and young adults.

16. Louis J. Novick, "How Traditional Judaism Helps the Aged Meet Their Psychological Needs," *Journal of Jewish Communal Service* 48, no. 3 (spring 1972): 286–94.

17. Kevin Kirkland and Howard McIlveen, *Full Circle: Spiritual Therapy for the Elderly* (New York and London: Haworth Press, 1999), xiii (citing Steve Atkinson, "Churchgoers Live Longer, Are Happier," *Nanaimo Daily News*, 4 July 1993, p. D7).

18. Cary Kozberg, "Let Your Heart Take Courage: A Ceremony for Entering a Nursing Home," in *A Heart of Wisdom: Making the Jewish Journey from Midlife through the Elder Years*," ed. Susan Berrin (Woodstock, Vt.: Jewish Lights Publishing, 1997), 289–97.

When Our Parents Can No Longer Decide

1. One such resource is Richard F. Address and the Commission on Jewish Family Concerns, eds., *A Time to Prepare: A Practical Guide for Individuals and Families in Determining a Jewish Approach to Making Personal*

Arrangements, Establishing the Limits of Medical Care, and Embracing Rituals at the End of Life, rev. ed. (New York: UAHC Press, 2002).

2. Rabbi Solomon Ganzfried, *Code of Jewish Law*, trans. Hyman E. Goldin (New York: Hebrew Publishing Company, 1963), 4:3.

3. Ibid., 3.

4. Benjamin Freedman, *Duty and Healing: Foundations of a Jewish Bioethic* (New York and London: Routledge, 1990), 122.

5. Ibid., 123.

6. Ganzfried, *Code*, 4:89.

On Suffering

1. Robert Gordis, *Kohelet: The Man and His World* (New York: Schocken Books, 1968 [1951]), 116.

2. Neil Gillman, *Sacred Fragments: Recovering Theology for the Modern Jew* (Philadelphia: Jewish Publication Society, 1990), 192.

3. Ibid., 193.

4. George Foot Moore, *Judaism in the First Centuries of the Christian Era* (New York: Schocken Books, 1971 [1927]), 1:547.

5. Solomon Schechter, *Aspects of Rabbinic Theology* (New York: Schocken Books, 1961 [1909]), 304–312.

6. Steven Schwarzschild, "Suffering," *Encyclopaedia Judaica*, 15:486.

7. David Hartman, *A Living Covenant: The Innovative Spirit in Traditional Judaism* (New York: The Free Press, 1985), especially chap. 8: "Rabbinic Responses to Suffering," 183–203; and David Hartman, "Suffering," in *Contemporary Jewish Religious Thought: Original Essays on Critical Concepts, Movements and Beliefs*, ed. Arthur A. Cohen and Paul Mendes-Flohr (New York: The Free Press, 1987), 939–46.

8. Hartman, "Suffering," 943–44.

9. Hartman, *A Living Covenant*, 195.

10. For a good summary of twentieth-century Jewish theologians' positions on suffering, see Gillman, *Sacred Fragments*, 198–211.

11. Richard Rubenstein, *After Auschwitz: Radical Theology and Contemporary Judaism* (Indianapolis: Bobbs-Merrill, 1966).

12. Harold Kushner, *When Bad Things Happen to Good People* (New York: Avon Books, 1981), 141, 146.

13. Ibid., 127–28.

14. Rabbi David Wolpe, *The Healer of Shattered Hearts* (New York: Henry Holt and Company, 1990), 159. Or read Rabbi Wolpe's more recent *Making Loss Matter: Creating Meaning in Difficult Times* (New York: Riverhead Books, 1999).

15. Rabbi Naomi Levy, *To Begin Again* (New York: Ballantine Books, 1998), 262.

16. Eric J. Cassell, "The Nature of Suffering," in *The Nature of Suffering and the Goals of Medicine* (New York: Oxford University Press, 1991), 44–45.

17. Rabbi Nachman of Bratslav, *Likutei Moharan Tinyana 11*, quoted in Aryeh Kaplan, *Meditation and Kabbalah* (York Beach, Maine: Samuel Weiser, 1982), 310.

Accepting Death: The Caregiver's Dilemma

1. So in the *El Malei Rachamim* prayer.

2. Significantly, the *Rabbi's Manual* contains only a Hebrew confession; the English translation is omitted—apparently it is deemed too distressing to speak and hear.

3. I have discussed this issue in a recent book, *The Price and Privilege of Growing Old* (New York: CCAR Press, 2000), 124–27.

Suggested Reading

Address, Richard F., ed. *A Time to Prepare*. New York: UAHC Press, 2001.

Aiken, Lisa. *Why Me God? A Jewish Guide for Coping and Suffering*. Northvale, N.J.: Jason Aronson, 1998.

Albom, Mitch. *Tuesdays With Morrie*. New York: Doubleday, 1997.

Amarnick, Claude. *Don't Put Me in a Nursing Home*. Palm Beach, Fla.: Garrett Publishing, 1996.

Berrin, Susan, ed. *A Heart of Wisdom: Making the Jewish Journey from Mid-Life Through the Elder Years*. Woodstock, Vt.: Jewish Lights Publishing, 1999.

Birren, James E., and K. Warner Schaie, eds. *Handbook of the Psychology of Aging*. San Diego: Academic Press, 2001.

Freeman, David, and Judith Z. Abrams. *Illness and Health in the Jewish Tradition: Writings from the Bible to Today*. Philadelphia: Jewish Publication Society, 1999.

Friedan, Betty. *The Fountain of Age*. New York: Simon & Schuster, 1993.

Friedman, Dayle A. *Jewish Pastoral Care: A Practical Handbook*. Woodstock, Vt.: Jewish Lights Publishing, 2001.

Hendershott, Anne B. *The Reluctant Caregivers: Learning to Care for a Loved One with Alzheimer's*. Westport, Conn.: Bergin and Garvey, 2000.

Hodgon, Harriet. *Alzheimer's—Finding the Words: A Communication Guide for Those Who Care*. New York: John Wiley & Sons, 1995.

Ilardo, Joseph A., and Carole R. Rothman. *Are Your Parents Driving You Crazy? How to Resolve the Most Common Dilemmas With Aging Parents*. Acton, Mass.: VanderWyk & Burnham, 2001.

Karpinski, Marion. *Quick Tips for Caregivers.* Medford, Oreg.: Healing Arts Communications, 2000.

Kaufmann, Sharon R. *The Ageless Self: Sources of Meaning in Late Life.* Madison, Wisc.: University of Wisconsin Press, 1994.

Kuhn, Daniel, and David A. Bennett. *Alzheimer's Early Stages: First Steps in Caring and Treatment.* Alameda, Calif.: Hunter House, 1999.

Lebow, Grace, Irwin Lebow, and Barbara Kane. *Coping with Your Difficult Older Parent: A Guide for Stressed-Out Children.* New York: Avon Books, 1999.

Loverde, Joy. *The Complete Eldercare Planner: Where to Start, Which Questions to Ask, and How to Find Help.* New York: Hyperion, 2000.

Masoro, Edward J., and Steen N. Austed, eds. *Handbook of the Biology of Aging.* San Diego: Academic Press, 2001.

McCleod, Beth Witrogen. *Caregiving: The Spiritual Journey of Love, Loss, and Renewal.* New York: John Wiley & Sons, 2000.

Morris, Virginia, and Robert Butler. *How to Care for Aging Parents.* New York: Workman Publishing Company, 1996.

Olitzky, Kerry M. *Jewish Paths Toward Healing and Wholeness: A Personal Spiritual Guide to Dealing with Suffering.* Jewish Lights Publishing, Woodstock, Vt., 2000.

Person, Hara E. *The Mitzvah of Healing.* New York: UAHC Press, 2003.

Riemer, Jack, and Nathaniel Stampfer. *So That Your Values Live On: Ethical Wills and How to Prepare Them.* Woodstock, Vt.: Jewish Lights Publishing, 1994.

Sales, Amy L. *Help, Opportunities, and Programs for Jewish Elders.* Waltham, Mass.: Cohen Center for Modern Jewish Studies, Brandeis University, 1998.

Silin, Peter S. *Nursing Homes: The Family's Journey.* Baltimore: Johns Hopkins University Press, 2001.

Sonsino, Rifat and Daniel B. Syme. *What Happens After I Die: Jewish Views of Life After Death.* New York: UAHC Press, 1990.

United Seniors Health Council. *Planning for Long Term Care.* New York: McGraw-Hill Trade, 2002.

Vaillant, George E. *Aging Well: Surprising Guideposts to a Happier Life from the Landmark Harvard Study of Adult Development.* London: Little, Brown & Company, 2002.

Wei, Jeanne, and Sue Levkoff. *Aging Well: The Complete Guide to Physical and Emotional Health.* New York: John Wiley & Sons, 2000.

Weintraub, Simkha Y. *Healing of Soul, Healing of Body: Spiritual Leaders Unfold the Strength and Solace in Psalms.* Woodstock, Vt.: Jewish Lights Publishing, 1994.

Contributors

 C& &D

RABBI RICHARD F. ADDRESS serves as the director of the Union of American Hebrew Congregations' Department of Jewish Family Concerns. Rabbi Address joined the UAHC staff in 1978 after pulpit work in California. He served as Regional Director of the Pennsylvania Council of the UAHC from August of 1978 through December of 2000. Ordained from Hebrew Union College–Jewish Institute of Religion (Cincinnati) in 1972, he received his honorary Doctor of Divinity from HUC-JIR in 1997. In 1998 he received a Certificate in Pastoral Counseling from the Post Graduate Center for Mental Health in New York and his Doctor of Ministry from the Hebrew Union College in New York in 1999. He is married to Jane Travis-Address and they have three children.

JANICE (JAN) LONDON BERGMAN is a native of Skokie, Illinois. She now resides outside of Washington, D.C., where she served with distinction for ten years as the Assistant Regional Director and the Regional Administrator of the UAHC Mid-Atlantic Council. She currently serves on the UAHC Jewish Family Concerns Committee, to which she brings firsthand experience in disability, aging, and mental health issues. In the past, Jan has also served as a volunteer leader on the boards of the Association for Retarded Citizens (the Arc) at the national, state, and local levels. When Jan moved her parents from Florida to the D.C. area, she was

immediately thrust into the "sandwich generation," adding to her responsibilities as the mother and stepmother of two young women with disabilities. Yet, with all the difficulties, she savors those last few years with her
mom and dad close by, knowing that their lives were enriched by the closeness of family. Her father died four weeks after her mother. She draws comfort from the idea that her parents are finally together again.

RABBI SANDRA ROSENTHAL BERLINER is the Director of Chaplaincy/
Rabbi of the Madlyn and Leonard Abramson Center for Jewish Life, in
Horsham, Pennsylvania. Previously, she directed the Jewish Hospice
Program of Philadelphia for twelve years, as well as serving a congrega-
tion in Philadelphia. Rabbi Berliner was a founding member of the
National Association of Jewish Chaplains and served as president of that
organization. She received her rabbinical ordination from the
Reconstructionist Rabbinical College, her M.S.W. from Case Western
Reserve University, School of Applied Social Sciences, and her B.A. from
Brandeis University.

RABBI MICHAEL CHERNICK is Deutsch Professor of Jewish Jurisprudence
and Social Justice at HUC-JIR/New York. He was educated at Yeshiva
College and Bernard Revel Graduate School and was ordained at Rabbi
Isaac Elchanan Theological Seminary. He specializes in Talmudic and
halachic literature.

RABBI DAYLE A. FRIEDMAN directs the Geriatric Chaplaincy Program at
the Reconstructionist Rabbinical College, where she is developing
Hiddur: the Center for Aging and Judaism. She edited *Jewish Pastoral
Care: A Practical Handbook from Traditional and Contemporary Sources*
(Woodstock, Vt.: Jewish Lights Publishing, 2001). She was the founding
Director of Chaplaincy Services at Philadelphia Geriatric Center from
1985 until 1997. She earned her rabbinic ordination at Hebrew Union
College–Jewish Institute of Religion, a Master's in Social Work from the
University of Southern California, and an M.A. in Jewish Communal
Service from Hebrew Union College.

RABBI ALAN HENKIN has served as Regional Director of the Pacific
Southwest Council of the Union of American Hebrew Congregations

since July 2000. Previously, he served as the rabbi for Temple Beth Solomon of the Deaf in Arleta, California, and then as rabbi of Congregation Beth Knesset Bamidbar in Lancaster, California. Rabbi Henkin was ordained by Hebrew Union College in Cincinnati in 1980, and he holds a Ph.D. in Social Ethics from the School of Religion at the University of Southern California, where he also earned an undergraduate degree. Rabbi Henkin has published articles in such journals as *The American Rabbi*, *The Jewish Spectator*, *The Journal of Reform Judaism*, *Judaism*, *The Reconstructionist*, and *Reform Judaism* and has taught at Hebrew Union College in Los Angeles. He was born in Chicago, Illinois, and is married to Susan Henkin, a registered nurse. They currently live in Northridge, California, and have four children.

KATHRYN KAHN has served for eight years as Associate National Director of Outreach and Synagogue Community in the William and Lottie Daniel Department of Outreach of the UAHC. She resides in Glen Ridge, New Jersey.

DR. ADINA KALET is an Assistant Professor of Medicine at the New York University School of Medicine. A primary care physician in New York City since 1984, she has a special interest in doctor-patient communication and studies, teaches, and publishes on this subject. An expert in the joy of balancing the personal and the professional, she works with her husband, also a physician. They live in Brooklyn with their two children, where they are members of the Park Slope Jewish Center.

DR. ROBERT L. KATZ, z"l, was Professor of Religion, Ethics, and Human Relations at Hebrew Union College–Jewish Institute of Religion in Cincinnati.

RABBI JONATHAN P. KENDALL was born in Youngstown, Ohio—the only son of Dr. Milton and Ann Kendall. He is a graduate of Ohio State University, where he majored in philosophy and linguistics. He is an ordinee of Hebrew Union College in Cincinnati, from which he recently received a Doctor of Divinity degree. Rabbi Kendall is the founding rabbi of Temple Beit HaYam in Stuart, Florida. He has served on state and local boards of HRS and the Department of Children and Families. He writes a biweekly column for Scripps-Howard newspapers and enjoys golf, boating, and windsurfing. He is the proud father of Jessica and Rivkah.

RABBI RUTH LANGER is Associate Professor of Jewish Studies in the Theology Department of Boston University, and Judaica Scholar at the Center for Christian Jewish Learning, Boston College. Ordained by Hebrew Union College–Jewish Institute of Religion in 1986, she received a Ph.D. from HUC-JIR in 1994. She is the author of numerous books and articles, including *To Worship God Properly: Tensions between Liturgical Custom and Halakhah in Judaism* (Cincinnati: Hebrew Union College Press, 1998).

DR. ALBERT MICAH LEWIS is the Director of the Aquinas Emeritus College. He is an Adjunct Professor of Jewish Studies at Michigan State University and Professor of Gerontology and Psychology at Aquinas College. Dr. Lewis is the Rabbi Emeritus of Congregation Emanuel in Grand Rapids, Michigan, former chairman of the CCAR Committee on Aging, and a weekly columnist for the *Grand Rapids Press* on issues of middle-aging and aging. With Jerome Folkman and Malcolm Stern, he was the co-author of *Retirement Begins at Forty*, published by the CCAR. He is the founding president of Hospice of Greater Grand Rapids and a frequent scholar in residence for UAHC congregations.

RABBI THOMAS A. LOUCHHEIM was ordained by Hebrew Union College–Jewish Institute of Religion in 1987. He is the rabbi of Congregation Or Chadash in Tucson, Arizona. He has served as the chaplain at the local Jewish nursing home and as the chairman of the CCAR Aging Committee. He has lectured on spiritual views of the afterlife, the role of suffering in ethical decision making, and the spiritual needs of caregivers to nurses, social workers, and clinicians.

RABBI SHELDON MARDER, ordained by Hebrew Union College in 1978, has been the spiritual leader of San Francisco's Jewish Home since 1999. He is experienced in the congregational rabbinate and in the field of higher Jewish education, having served as Director of the Rabbinic School and Associate Dean of HUC in Los Angeles. He studies and teaches modern Hebrew poetry and the Book of Psalms. He and his wife,

Rabbi Janet Marder, are the parents of two daughters—Betsy and Rachel. His parents, Frances and Jack, are residents of the Jewish Home.

RABBI HARA E. PERSON is the Editorial Director of the UAHC Press. Ordained by Hebrew Union College–Jewish Institute of Religion in 1998, she holds a B.A. from Amherst College and a M.A. in Fine Arts from New York University/International Center of Photography. She lives in Brooklyn, New York, with her husband and children.

RABBI DEBORAH PIPE-MAZO is the Director of Rabbinic Services for the Central Conference of American Rabbis. Ordained by Hebrew Union College, New York Campus, in 1991, she is a certified chaplain in the National Association of Jewish Chaplains. She lives and works from her home in Barnstable, Massachusetts, is married to Rabbi Gary Mazo, and has three children, Ari, Daniel, and Sara.

RABBI W. GUNTHER PLAUT is the editor of the groundbreaking *The Torah: A Modern Commentary* and *The Haftarah Commentary*, both published by the UAHC Press. He is also the co-editor, along with Michael A. Meyer, of *The Reform Judaism Reader* and is the author of numerous other books and articles. Having served for many years as the rabbi of Holy Blossom Temple in Toronto, Ontario, he is now the Senior Scholar of Holy Blossom Temple.

HARRIET HOLLANDER ROSEN has a long involvement in Jewish communal organizations and is an active member of the UAHC Jewish Family Concerns Committee. She and her husband, Gil, live in Scottsdale, Arizona, and are blessed with two daughters, two sons-in-law, and three grandchildren—and all of them are blessed by her parents' memory.

DR. JAMES SOFFER is a dentist from Cherry Hill, New Jersey. He met his wife, Bess, at UAHC Camp Harlam, where he is currently chairman of the camp committee. They have two sons. He is a lifelong member of Temple Emanuel, Cherry Hill, New Jersey.

LAURA SPERLING received a bachelor's degree in Ethnomusicology and World Arts Culture from UCLA. She has performed both Western and non-Western repertoire as a soloist and with various chamber music ensembles in Los Angeles and Seattle and has performed throughout the United States. In 1994 and 1995, Ms. Sperling made concert appearances in the Ukraine region of the former Soviet Union and has made annual appearances in Mexico since 1996. Ms. Sperling teaches flute and recorder and has developed and teaches an early childhood music program, The Imagination Express. She has released her first CD, *Water Music*, for solo flutes. This CD includes Ms. Sperling's performance on the Japanese porcelain flute, which she has designed and helped to create.

RABBI JACK STERN is Rabbi Emeritus of Westchester Reform Temple in Scarsdale, New York, where he served from 1962 until his retirement in 1991. He is a past president of the Central Conference of American Rabbis and currently chairs the CCAR Committee on Ethics and Procedures and Guidelines. He resides in Great Barrington, Massachusetts, where he is a member of Hevreh of Southern Berkshire.

RABBI DAVID WOLFMAN is the Regional Director of the UAHC Northeast Council and is the Director of the National Commission on Rabbi Congregational Relations. He received his B.A. in Sociology and Religion from Boston University and attended rabbinical school at Hebrew Union College–Jewish Institute of Religion, where he received his M.A.H.L. and was ordained rabbi. He lives in Lexington, Massachusetts, with his wife, three daughters, and his grandmother-in-law.